Your Menopause

Myra Hunter is a clinical psychologist specialising in women's health. She has counselled menopausal women for many years and, at Kings College Hospital in London, set up a project to investigate how women are really affected by the menopause. Her findings were published to international acclaim and established her as the leading researcher in the field. Myra Hunter lives in London with her husband and twin daughters.

Your Menopause

Prepare now for a positive future

MYRA HUNTER

PANDORA

LONDON   SYDNEY   WELLINGTON

First published in 1990 by Pandora Press, an imprint of the Trade
Division of Unwin Hyman Ltd

Pandora Press
Unwin Hyman Limited
15/17 Broadwick Street,
London W1V 1FP

Unwin Hyman Inc
8 Winchester Place, Winchester, MA 01890, USA

Allen & Unwin Australia Pty Ltd
PO Box 764, 8 Napier Street, North Sydney, NSW 2060, Australia

Allen & Unwin New Zealand Pty Ltd with the Port Nicholson Press
Compusales Building, 75 Ghuznee Street, Wellington, New Zealand

British Library Cataloguing in Publication Data
Hunter, Myra
  Your menopause.
  1. Women. Menopause
  I. Title
  612'.665

ISBN 0-04-440625-8

Typeset in 11 on 13 point Bembo by
Input Typesetting Ltd, London SW19 8DR
Printed in Finland by Werner Söderström Oy

For My Mother

Acknowledgements

Thanks first to the hundreds of women who took part in my research and who took the time to describe their experiences before, during and after the menopause. I also learned a lot from those who faced problems during the menopause and came to see me, as well from the staff of the Menopause Clinic at King's College Hospital. I am especially grateful to Sheila Lawler for her help in typing the manuscript, to Candida Lacey at Pandora, for her advice and constructive criticism and, finally, to my husband Jim for his valuable comments as well as his support and encouragement.

Contents

Introduction

The menopause is part of a woman's *normal* development and refers specifically to her last menstrual period. But the menopause is a taboo subject for men *and* for women: it is rarely discussed seriously or openly and instead it is a source of embarrassment, jokes, fear and confusion. Few people know enough about or really understand the menopause, and menopausal women are the butt of powerful prejudices that combine both sexism and ageism.

The current view, which is supported by the medical profession and the media, is of the menopause as a deficiency disease. This means that women are deficient in the hormone oestrogen after the menopause. Oestrogen deficiency means decline and deterioration of skin, bones and other bodily systems, rapid ageing and reduced sexual enjoyment. Is this really what we have to look forward to?

By the mid-1990s approximately seven million women in Britain will be menopausal or will have recently experienced menopause. These women will represent an increasing proportion of the population and, because of the general decline in birth rates and the postwar baby-boom, this will be the case until the end of the century. And now that the average life expectancy for women is 78, we can hope to spend a third of our lives after the menopause.

Contrary to popular belief, this *can* be a very positive time of life.

If you are aged 30 or over, you are part of the generation of women who sought, or who are seeking, information and active participation in pregnancy and childbirth. You set out to explore and learn about women's sexuality, fertility and contraception, and related health problems. Having fought for, and won, more opportunities and independence in your twenties and thirties, surely you don't want to look forward to several decades of decline?

In my experience many younger women tend not to *think* about this stage in life, but they may have general feelings of foreboding about it – which are usually negative and sometimes frightening. This attitude of denial differs considerably from the active approach that many women take when anticipating childbirth. The advantages of being informed about changes during labour, of keeping to a healthy diet and the benefits of particular techniques that can make childbirth easier are now generally acknowledged. The menopause has been largely neglected by feminists and people who are concerned about women's health. It is one of the last remaining major health issues to be tackled.

In this book I want to encourage women to think positively about their menopause and *prepare* for it. By seeking information and questioning established attitudes you can help to change your own views and face the future with confidence. You can also begin to make family, friends and colleagues both at home and at work more aware. By taking care about exercise and diet you can help to prevent specific problems from occurring. By being better informed and by anticipating events you can regain control of the menopause, as well as general life changes which may occur at the same time. Preparation will enable you to make the right choices about available treatments and to know where to seek help if you need to.

Here are some of the most common questions women ask about the menopause:

- What will I experience during and after the menopause?
- Are these changes caused by biological factors, or ageing, or general life changes?
- Is the menopause a natural event – part of normal development – or is it a medical problem?
- What treatments are available that are safe and effective?
- Are there alternatives to hormone replacement therapy (HRT)?
- What can I do to prepare for the menopause?

I was repeatedly asked such questions when, as a clinical psychologist in a London teaching hospital, I worked with menopausal women for eight years. Women who sought medical help because they were depressed or generally unwell, were often confused about their symptoms. They were unsure about whether these problems could be attributed to the menopause, and often their doctors were too. I examined the research which was available to find the answers, but to no avail. So *I* decided to carry out a large study to explore the experiences of ordinary women, both before and after the menopause.

In the 1980s large scale studies were set up: two in North America – by Patricia Kaufert in Manitoba, Canada[1] and in Massachusetts by Sonja and John McKinlay[2] – one in Norway led by Arne Holte,[3] and my own study of women living in South East England.[4] Unlike earlier studies (which relied upon samples of women who attended a doctor or clinic or compared women of different ages), we sampled large numbers of ordinary women and then followed a proportion of them through their menopause for between three and five years. Only in this way can the nature of changes during the menopause be understood.

I have counselled many women who had problems during the menopause, including women who experienced premature menopause, either naturally or as a result of surgery or disease. In addition, I have spoken to many women individually, in groups and at workshops. Throughout this book I will draw on their experiences as well as the results of the research studies, in an attempt to provide a more balanced picture of the menopause.

Attitudes towards menopausal women are unnecessarily negative and changing these attitudes will be a major task. The 'deficiency disease' view of the menopause implies that *all* menopausal women are either ill or deficient – unless they undergo oestrogen therapy (HRT). This image of menopausal women is detrimental to women's self-esteem and encourages the pessimism that surrounds this period of life. It is not that I am against oestrogen therapy; it may clearly be the solution for some women. For others, however, it is not the answer.

This book will help *you* to decide what is best for *you*. During the years I have worked with menopausal women I have found that the menopause need not be a crisis and that we need to develop more positive attitudes and expectations. It is vital that women have up-to-date information if we are to prepare properly for this stage of our lives. I hope that this book will provide you with the information you need to make crucial decisions and to prepare for the future.

1

The Menopause

WHAT IS IT?

Most women remember when and where they started their first period. Many women expect the end of their fertile phase of life to be an equally sudden and obvious event. It might be a lot easier if this were the case. But it is not.

> I admit I've got mixed feelings about the menopause. I've missed a couple of periods and last time I disposed of my tampons, but now I'm having another period. Not knowing whether I've gone through the menopause or not is like waiting for something terrible to happen – I think I'll feel better when this transitional phase is over.

The *menopause*, from the Greek meaning month and cessation, literally means your last menstrual period. Every woman must go through it – provided she lives long enough – although a small number will experience it prematurely, as a result of surgery or disease.

The World Health Organisation defines the menopause as, 'permanent cessation of menstruation resulting from loss of ovarian follicular activity'. But another term – *climacteric* (which is also used) – has a much broader meaning: it takes in the whole period of gradual reduction in ovulation and the decrease in the output of hormones from the ovaries. Climacteric is largely a medical term, derived from a Greek word meaning a critical phase. The World Health Organisation defines the climacteric as, 'The period immediately prior to the menopause (when the endocrinological, biological and clinical features of approaching menopause commence) and at least the first year after the menopause.'

So the climacteric describes the years spanning the transition between reproductive and non-reproductive life, but there is little agreement about when it begins and how long it lasts. Estimates vary between ten and fifteen years, starting usually between the ages of 40 and 55. The phrases 'climacteric syndrome' and 'climacteric symptoms' are often used by doctors to describe a wide variety of physical and emotional complaints. The trouble with these labels is that really any problem can be attributed to the climacteric or menopause for a considerable number of years.

The menopause itself can be divided into stages which are all determined by the patterns of your menstrual periods: *Premenopausal* – when you are menstruating regularly; *Perimenopausal* – your menstruation has become irregular but has occurred during the previous twelve months; and *Postmenopausal* – you have not menstruated for at least twelve months.

The medical assessment of the menopause – in other words whether you are menopausal or not – usually relies on this classification. In addition hormones, usually oestrogen, which every woman has in her body can be measured by blood tests to determine whether you are pre- or postmenopausal.

However the colloquial phrase 'the change of life' refers not just to menstrual and hormonal changes but it includes many physical, emotional, social and general life changes which may occur in midlife. And 'menopausal syndrome' is a term which is also frequently used. But this is misleading because it suggests that there are more symptoms associated with the menopause than is actually the case. The symptoms listed by doctors in medical literature include: hot flushes, night sweats (known as vasomotor symptoms); vaginal changes, including thinning of vaginal wall and dryness; poor memory, loss of concentration; osteoporosis (thinning of the bones); depression, anxiety, irritability, loss of libido, tension; and many physical symptoms, such as insomnia, headaches, dry skin and hair, weight gain, dizziness, tiredness, palpitations, aching limbs and joints, itchiness and loss of energy.

It is true to say that hot flushes, night sweats and vaginal dryness are the most characteristic physical sensations of the peri- and postmenopausal stages. But the other symptoms or possible changes should *not* be included as part of the menopause automatically. The use of such a loose term as 'menopausal syndrome' is not at all helpful to women – they want explanations and understanding about themselves and their bodily changes.

WHEN WILL IT HAPPEN?

The *average* age for onset of the menopause is between 50 and 51 years. Generally there is surprising consistency in the average age at which menstruation stops across the world. Of course, there are small variations. In Britain it is 49.75 years, in the United States it is estimated as 51.4 years. Although most people link the menopause with the fiftieth year, few realise that it can occur quite normally during a *wide* age-range – at any time between 40 and 60. When it occurs before the age of 40 it is usually considered *premature*.

It is difficult to predict when the menopause will occur. There is often a strong family pattern in the timing – ask your mother, grandmothers, elder sisters and aunts to provide some clues. There does seem to be a tendency for it to come earlier in women who smoke and slightly later in overweight women. Other factors such as age at menarche (onset of menstruation), age at last pregnancy, if you have used oral contraceptives and how many times you were pregnant have been found to influence with the timing of the menopause by some researchers – but not by others.

When the menopause happens can be very important. I have found that women who experience 'early' menopause tend to report greater physical discomfort and emotional distress largely because they are unprepared. Whether you describe your menopause as premature or not may partly depend upon your expectations of when it *should* occur. But I imagine that most women would be surprised to undergo the menopause in their thirties or early forties.

An early menopause can bring women face to face with issues of fertility – it may even be that pregnancies have been planned 'at some time in the future'. So fertility seems to be less of an issue for women experiencing menopause in their late forties and early fifties. Early menopause can also result from surgery, such as the removal of the ovaries (oophorectomy), or disease, such as ovarian cancer, as well as treatments, such as certain drugs used to treat cancer and some forms of radiotherapy. It is worth consulting your doctor if your periods stop for several months because early menopause is easily diagnosed.

Mary became menopausal in her late twenties after a hysterectomy and the removal of her ovaries. This was done because she suffered from endometriosis (the growth of the lining of the womb around the ovaries, which causes pain. For more information contact the Endometriosis Society page 165.) She said, 'I felt cheated out of fertility at first. I'm gradually adjusting to it and we're now hoping to adopt a baby.'

Janet had her menopause in her mid-twenties following radiotherapy to treat Hodgkin's disease. She is not married: 'The worst thing is not being given an explanation or information beforehand. The hot flushes came as a shock and I felt very depressed for months. Now I'm on HRT [hormone replacement therapy] I feel better. But I do feel awkward and embarrassed about telling people I don't have periods and that I can't have children.'

Susan, 36, had her menopause in her early thirties for no obvious reason. 'Sam and I have been together for years. When the option was taken away I desperately wanted children, although we'd not been keen on a family before. My friends began to offer me time with their children which I found very insensitive.'

I will discuss early menopause and all that that implies on pages 39 and 82. At the same time, a late menopause may be welcomed by some women and disliked by others. Some women who continue to have menstrual periods into their late fifties find it irritating and inconvenient.

WHY DOES IT HAPPEN?

Hormone Changes

The menopause is triggered off by hormonal changes. To make sense of what happens to your hormones during the menopause, you need to understand the changes that take place during a menstrual cycle (see page 8 for diagram).

The Menstrual Cycle

Around 2 to 5 million eggs (or follicles) already exist in your ovaries at birth. The numbers gradually reduce, so by the time you are eleven there are about 500,000. Some eggs die, and after puberty one or sometimes two eggs are released each month.

The menstrual cycle is governed by hormones, which are sent directly into the bloodstream from the ovaries, as well as from the adrenal glands (situated above the kidneys). There are at least three different kinds of hormones, the main ones being oestrogens and progestins. Androgens are also produced in small quantities.

The ovaries and adrenals are given chemical messages by the pituitary gland, at the base of the brain. The pituitary gland releases follicle stimulating hormone (FSH) and leuteinising hormone (LH). These hormones trigger the ovaries to put out oestrogen and progesterone, and in turn the levels of oestrogen and progesterone in the bloodstream regulate the amounts of FSH and LH secreted. So a feedback mechanism balances the amounts of hormones during the menstrual cycle.

During the first part of the cycle FSH causes the egg to mature or ripen and the oestrogen levels rise. Ovulation, when the egg leaves the ovaries, is triggered when oestrogen reaches a certain level in the bloodstream and causes the pituitary to produce a wave of LH. The egg is released into the fallopian tube and, if it is not fertilised, it passes out of the womb. The egg leaves a scar on the ovary, called the corpus luteum, which makes oestrogen and progesterone. These hormones continue to thicken the lining of the womb (or endometrium). If pregnancy does not occur the corpus luteum disintegrates, which causes levels of oestrogen and progesterone to fall and then the lining of the womb is shed. Menstruation then occurs and the whole cycle begins again.

Few women really follow the textbook twenty-eight day pattern, with five days of bleeding and ovulation on day fourteen. There are enormous variations between women and between months.

The Menopause

During the forty years or so of having periods about 500 eggs will have reached maturity. It is estimated that by your mid-forties you have about 8,000 eggs left. Two important things happen before the menopause – a gradual stopping of ovulation and a decline in the output of oestrogen by the ovaries.

An important point to remember is that it is still possible to become pregnant for at least a year after the last menstrual period, so contraceptives are still necessary for two years if you are under 50 and for one year if you are over 50.

As the menopause approaches the feedback mechanism between the ovaries and the pituitary gland which I mentioned before is upset and, as a result, FSH and LH levels in the blood begin to rise. It is as if these hormones are working overtime to try to trigger some action from the

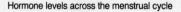
Hormone levels across the menstrual cycle

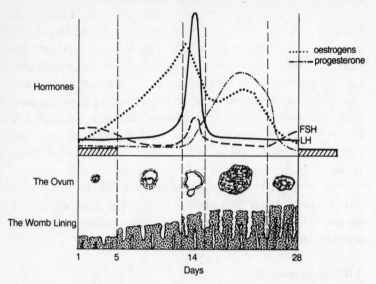

ovaries to produce hormones. There is an earlier and greater rise in FSH than LH. FSH levels are at their highest three to five years after the menopause and then they return to premenopausal levels. LH levels rise, but not so dramatically, until about five years after the menopause and then they reduce again. The blood test used by doctors to determine whether you are menopausal or not usually detects rises in FSH, as well as lowered oestrogen levels, because these are the early biological signs of the onset of the menopause.

During and after the menopause there are changes in the production of oestrogen and progesterone. Usually these are measured in the bloodstream. But the *relationship* between them is as important as their *rate* of change. There are several types of oestrogens. During the reproductive years the major one is oestradiol which is produced by the ovary. After the menopause, oestrogen supplies *do not stop*, because another oestrogen called oestrone is produced from three major sources: the adrenal cortex in the adrenal gland; indirectly from the body's fat cells which convert another hormone (androstenedione) to oestrone; and from the ovaries (unless you have had them surgically removed), which continue to manufacture small quantities of androgens which are converted to oestrogens.

After the menopause about 85 per cent of oestrogens circulating in the bloodstream are produced by the adrenals and 15 per cent by the ovaries. There is a lot of variation between women in the amounts of hormones present through the years before, during and after the menopause, and one reason for this is that higher levels of oestrogen are produced in those who have more body fat.

If you experience a natural menopause your hormones are likely to adjust gradually, while if you have a surgically-induced menopause there is a more dramatic change in the hormone levels – often producing more symptoms.

Another hormone, progesterone, is associated with the premenstrual phase in the menstrual cycle. Progesterone levels decrease before and during the menopause but again the adrenal glands continue to secrete small amounts afterwards.

Finally testosterone remains at the same level after the menopause. It is produced by the adrenal glands and by the conversion of other hormones.

Much about the intricate relationship between these hormones is still not understood. Given the upsurges in LH and FSH and the readjustment in production of hormones, it would be surprising if we were unaware of these changes in our bodies, or if we did not experience exaggerated menstrual symptoms at certain times. Bodily changes do occur but be in tune with them – you can *help* your body to adapt!

Hysterectomy and Surgical Menopause

Hysterectomy means removal of the womb. On its own this does *not* lead to premature menopause. Monthly periods cease but oestrogen levels in the body remain roughly the same.

The operation can be total (womb and cervix) or subtotal (leaving the cervix) and can be performed via the abdomen or the vagina. Hysterectomy is usually used as a remedy for cancer, fibroids, heavy bleeding or pelvic pain.

The number of hysterectomies has increased in recent years: in a survey of over 2,000 European women, aged between 40 and 70, 11 per cent had undergone a hysterectomy. There were differences between countries – 13.2 per cent in Britain, 15.5 per cent in Italy and 8.5 per cent in France[1] – but these figures are appreciably lower than those for the USA and Australia, where twice as many hysterectomies are carried out.

Estimates vary (although they are always relatively high) about the percentage of hysterectomies that are classifiable as 'unnecessary surgery'. There is some suggestion that the figure may be related to the race and social class of the women and whether or not they have medical insurance.[2]

Like the menopause, hysterectomy has been surrounded by mystery and fear. Many women expect a hysterectomy to lead to depression or sexual problems. Obviously the reasons for having the hysterectomy in the first place and how ill you are beforehand, as well as your general life circumstances, will influence your reactions to the operation.

A woman who has had her womb removed will experience menopause, possibly with hot flushes, at an age similar to other women. However there is some suggestion that those who have had a hysterectomy might have a slightly earlier menopause.

Oophorectomy or removal of the ovaries is an entirely separate operation – although sometimes it is performed simultaneously with a hysterectomy – and it *does* induce menopause. If you are having a hysterectomy it is very important to be clear about the difference between this operation and oophorectomy.

If you need a hysterectomy operation and have been adequately informed about it and have been given time to think and discuss the issues beforehand, then the operation may well not affect you. The decision to have a hysterectomy should only be taken with adequate time, information and discussion. There is certainly evidence showing that women who do not have negative expectations about the operation[3] and who are fully prepared make a better recovery.[4] If you are unsure as to whether you really need a hysterectomy or oophorectomy you should seek a second opinion. It is advisable, if at all possible, to keep your ovaries in order to prevent premature menopause. For details of hysterectomy support groups see page 165, and early menopause see pages 39, 82 and 146.

HOW LONG DOES IT LAST?

Again, women vary appreciably. If we think about the beginning of the menopause as the first changes in the menstrual cycle, and the ending as the last hot flushes, then it takes an average of between two and five years. However, given the enormously different experiences of women in all aspects of the menopause, it is vital that you do not view yourself as abnormal if the age, extent or nature of your menopause is not the same for you as it is for your friends, or if it is not consistent with the textbooks.

HOW DO YOU KNOW IT IS THE MENOPAUSE?

If you are trying to fit yourself into one of the categories or stages of the menopause and you are having difficulty, it's not surprising. Although the menopause is strictly defined by menstrual cycle changes, remember that hormonal fluctuations – possibly associated with hot flushes – begin *before* the last menstrual period. When I ask women whether they have started their menopause or not – and if so how do they know – the most common responses seem to be: My periods are irregular; I'm having hot flushes; I'm approaching fifty.

I suppose I ought to be menopausal in view of my age [49]. Although my periods seem to have lessened, with a heavier second day, they continue regularly every twenty-four to twenty-seven days.

My periods are heavier and now more frequent [twenty-two day cycle] than they were, so I think this is the beginning of the change.

My periods stopped for a year and I am now in the

process of having another period! So I'm confused. I hope that this is my last.

I have had irregular periods and I went to my doctor to find out if it was the menopause. He said that it probably is, so I'll just wait and see what happens next.

I'm sure I've gone through the menopause because my periods stopped just like that a year ago.

I think I'm starting the menopause because I've had slight irregularity recently and occasional night sweats.

The trouble with the menopause is that you can only really know that you have gone through it after the event – at least one year *after* your last menstrual period – because any period could be your last. The medical definitions all assume that you menstruate regularly and do not have spells of amenorrhea (no periods at all), which are quite common. Women I have talked to describe themselves as beginning the menopause when periods become irregular, that is *before* they have stopped altogether.

The way menstruation stops varies considerably – abruptly, gradually or irregularly. Some women report periods becoming lighter, others miss periods, before stopping altogether. Irregular cycles are the most common way for periods to cease; they may become closer together, further apart, heavier or lighter, and without a consistent pattern from month to month. Some months may be missed altogether. This unpredictability can be unpleasant for some women, and one way to feel more in control – and gain an overview of these changes and any hot flushes – is to keep a daily record (see Menstrual Diary).

Menstrual Diary

	1	2	3	4	5	6	7	8	9	10	11	12	13	14	15	16	17	18	19	20	21	22	23	24	25	26	27	28	29	30	31
Jan																															
Feb																															
Mar																															
Apr																															
May																															
Jun																															
Jul																															
Aug																															
Sep																															
Oct																															
Nov																															
Dec																															

X – periods
HF – hot flushes

It might be useful to note down any stressful events in the month – domestic crises, problems at work or moving house. This is because menstrual patterns and hot flushes can be sensitive to stress and disruption.

The menstrual patterns of 324 women, aged forty-five and over, were followed for a period of three years in a study carried out by Pat Kaufert and colleagues at the University of Manitoba, Canada.[5] The women were interviewed on six separate occasions and asked to chart their menstrual cycles. Some women went from regular periods to irregular periods and back again, and others stopped menstruating, started and stopped again. Only 12 per cent said that they were menstruating regularly at all six interviews. The researchers also studied the factors that might predict that there would be a change in a woman's menstrual pattern: 'Information that a patient has vasomotor symptoms [hot flushes and night sweats] or is depressed or irritable *does not* indicate the imminent approach of the menopause. Knowing a woman's age, her current pattern of menstruation and whether she has experienced menstrual flooding is more useful when calculating the odds on menstrual change.' Therefore changes in menstrual periods, age and heavy bleeding characterise 'the change' to a greater extent than emotional or other physical symptoms.

Quite naturally, at times you might be unsure whether some symptoms are normal or whether any indicate gynaecological problems or underlying illness. It can be reassuring to seek medical advice to exclude physical illness, and examination of hormone levels can clarify whether you are pre- or postmenopausal. Symptoms like irregular bleeding and flooding, or heavy bleeding, can be worrying. It is worth checking particularly if you have: bleeding which is very frequent (every two to three weeks); staining or spotting which occur for a week or more between periods; very heavy bleeding indeed (diffi-

cult to absorb with tampons or sanitary towels); bleeding
when the menopause is definitely over, that is when you
have not had periods for about a year. These symptoms
might not be serious and not require treatment. Polyps
(small growths in the cervix) and fibroids (growths of the
fibrous tissue in the uterus) are quite common and can
cause irregular or heavy bleeding. Polyps are easily
removed if necessary; fibroids usually shrink and often
disappear after the menopause, although they can also be
removed. But irregular bleeding can be the first warning
sign of cancer, which can be treated with early detection.
So do not put off seeking medical advice – take control,
and investigate the problem.

While it is quite common to have a few heavy periods
during the perimenopause, a small proportion of women
experience heavy periods in their thirties and forties.
Heavy periods, or menorrhagia, can be very inconvenient
and distressing, as this woman found. 'Every month I had
to go to bed for a week, no amount of towels could stop
the flow if I was standing up. I felt like a social outcast. I
had to leave my job.'

The most common causes of excessive bleeding are the
overstimulation of the womb by your natural hormones
or fibroids or a malignant growth. Your doctor will probably give you a pelvic examination, a cervical smear test
and possibly a dilatation and curettage (D and C). A small
area of the surface of the womb is removed. This in itself
can stop the bleeding or it can reveal any signs of cancer
of the womb.

If the bleeding is caused by hormone changes you will
probably be offered drug treatment, either a progestogen
(a synthetic progesterone) or Danozol (a drug which gre-
atly reduces bleeding and may stop periods altogether),

and these methods can be quite successful. If the cause is fibroids then these can be removed, but if they are very large, if you have cancer of the womb, or if bleeding is severe with no obvious cause, then you might be advised to have a hysterectomy. However, it might be worth trying vitamin and mineral supplements first because some women have been helped by ensuring that they have adequate supplies of vitamin A, iron and calcium, and people also claim that Efamol (evening primrose oil) relieves these symptoms.

Some women find that premenstrual tension (PMT) becomes worse during the years leading up to the menopause. Seventy-five per cent of premenopausal women usually say that they have suffered from PMT at some time, but when daily diaries are used to record menstrual periods and mood changes it seems that there is sometimes not such a clear link between mood changes and the premenstrual phase. Try it yourself to find out about your moods and your menstrual cycle.

But a number of women do describe considerable changes in emotional and physical feelings before their periods while they feel 'normal' the rest of the time. Given the hormonal upheavals which occur prior to the menopause it is perhaps not surprising that some women experience PMT for the first time, or that symptoms get worse before the menopause. Don't despair if you find that this happens to you – there is a great deal that you can do to alleviate the tension and deal with variations in general well-being. Vitamin B6 and, again, Efamol are popular remedies. These will be discussed further in the chapters that follow.

Menopausal Symptoms

Apart from the changes in the menstrual cycle, the main signs of the beginning of the menopausal process are physical symptoms, in particular hot flushes and night sweats. Some women also experience vaginal dryness after the menopause, which can make sexual activity uncomfortable. It is important to remember that these symptoms are the only symptoms that are definitely associated with the menopause, that they are not signs of disease and that there are several ways of alleviating them.

One health problem that is more common in older postmenopausal women is osteoporosis (thinning of the bones). For more about osteoporosis and ways of preventing it, see pages 54, 104, 113 and 137.

Hot Flushes

I have one or two hot flushes each week but they're quite normal aren't they?

I feel exhausted all the time. The night sweats are harder to cope with than the hot flushes because they disturb my sleep. The tiredness makes me feel low and less able to manage ordinary life. It's a vicious circle. My friends and family are urging me to see my GP and I think I'll have to now.

My hot flushes lasted about three years on and off, sometimes I had to go outside to cool down but they didn't really bother me.

I am thinking of having HRT (hormone replacement therapy) because I will be in the public eye making speeches, and I would be embarrassed to have hot flushes, otherwise I don't think I would consider HRT.

Hot flushes or flashes (as they are sometimes called) are usually described as hot sensations in the face, neck and chest which last a minute or two and are followed by a chill feeling or perspiration. While they may be intense for some women, they are *not* harmful, they do not cause physical damage and they will eventually stop. Unfortunately they can be embarrassing and disrupt sleep, as these experiences show.

It seems that about three-quarters of menopausal women experience hot flushes for over a year; approximately half may have them for two to five years, and they might continue for more than five years in about a quarter of women. Similarly about one in five women is unlikely to have hot flushes at all. This is thought to be the result of the higher levels of circulating oestrogen in some women, which are partly determined by body weight.

You might experience increased heart rate or palpitations at the onset of a hot flush, which can sometimes be misinterpreted as a sign of anxiety. One woman who had previously suffered from anxiety and panic attacks was worried about this sensation: 'When my hot flushes began I thought that my old symptoms were coming back again. It's reassuring to know that it's quite normal. I just sit down, relax and the palpitations go away.'

In one of the few studies in which women have been asked in detail about the experience of their flushes, Ann Voda, working at the University of Utah, interviewed and monitored twenty women over a fortnight.[6] The frequency and severity varied enormously – they reported having had between two and 247 hot flushes during the two-week period; night-time and daytime flushes were equally common and although the average length of hot flushes was three minutes, they ranged from thirty seconds to sixty minutes in length. Different parts of the body were affected: the face and neck were the most common but the lower parts of the body became hot in about half the women. Some flushes spread upwards and some downwards. More than half were rated as mild, a third as moderate and about 10 per cent as severe. When they were asked how they coped these women either did nothing or found practical ways to cool down, such as showering, opening a window or using a fan.

Many women I have spoken to get to know what might bring on a hot flush. These two women noticed the following links:

Whenever I get het up at work and am rushing around I get more hot flushes.

I certainly have more when it's hot – in the summer or in a strongly heated room – and sometimes if I drink a lot of coffee they come on.

You might experience hot flushes before the menopause when you are menstruating regularly. Some of the younger women (aged 25 to 35) I spoke to had experienced hot flushes before. These can occur at particular phases of the menstrual cycle. I remember having a few hot flushes during the days immediately after childbirth and this gives us a clue as to what might cause them.

It seems that they occur as a result of a *reduction* in oestrogen levels. But this does *not* mean that there is a direct relationship between oestrogen and hot flushes.

They seem to happen during the transition between higher and lower levels and they stop when the body has readjusted. Although the precise causes of hot flushes are not known, they are associated with surges of LH (leuteinising hormone) which may dilate the surface blood vessels.

Hot flushes are one of the symptoms that are alleviated by oestrogen therapy (HRT). When you stop treatment they can return for several months. For more about hot flushes and night sweats and how to deal with them, see pages 35 and 121.

Vaginal Changes
Most women know about the link between hot flushes and the menopause but only a few are aware that vaginal changes can also occur during and after the menopause. Vaginal dryness can be difficult to discuss, and it is frequently misunderstood. The women I talk to often mention vaginal dryness, but they generally do not regard it as a major problem. Just as with other symptoms, experiences of and reactions to vaginal dryness vary:

I didn't mind the hot flushes and was pleased about not having periods. It was the dryness of my vagina that was most difficult to deal with.

I didn't realise until the doctor explained that the dryness was part of the menopause. I thought that my feelings must have changed towards my husband.

I'm too embarrassed to tell the doctor, but I use KY jelly, and that helps.

I have to be more relaxed and aroused before penetration, and I find that a lubricant helps.

The vagina is one of the principal organs that uses oestrogen. After the menopause there are gradual changes in and around the vagina, but not all women experience this. The vaginal wall becomes thinner and loses some of its elasticity. This can produce a sensation of dryness and, if care is not taken, pain during intercourse. Vaginal infections or irritations may also become more common.

Dryness does respond to oestrogen treatment but alternative practical approaches are also available. If you have an active sexual life before the menopause or regularly masturbate, that is your vagina is regularly lubricated, you are less likely to experience dryness after the menopause. Turn to pages 124 and 137 for a full discussion on ways to cope with this.

The somewhat vague and intangible nature of the menopause – how it begins and ends, its indeterminate length and women's wide-ranging experiences – means that it is particularly prone to misunderstanding and stereotyping. And a common tendency is to attribute problems to the menopause which have other causes and solutions. Unfortunately negative images of menopausal women are still the rule rather than the exception.

2

Myths and Stereotypes

What images come to mind when you hear the word menopause?

How would you feel if you were called menopausal?

Can you openly talk about the menopause with your family, friends or at work?

WHAT DO YOU REALLY THINK ABOUT THE MENOPAUSE?

Like any taboo subject the menopause is rarely discussed seriously or directly. Instead vague terms are used like 'the change', 'midlife crisis' or 'change of life'. When the menopause is openly referred to the most common reaction is embarrassment or laughter. Why should the menopause be seen as amusing? Stereotypes about menopausal women are almost always negative in western countries. You may be characterised as over-emotional, aggressive, irrational, insane or depressed; you may be accused of being sexually disinterested or sexually over-aroused: a no-win situation. Not only that, you will probably be told that you are beginning to decline physically and will rapidly enter old age. The words and phrases used, particularly by the medical profession, clearly convey a catastrophic image of the menopause.

We are described as having:

- hormone deficiency
- vaginal atrophy
- ovarian failure
- loss of femininity
- empty nest syndrome
- rapidly thinning bones

These terms are all unnecessarily negative. In a culture that puts a high value upon youth and beauty, the menopause becomes an inferior state marking the beginning of old age. Robert Wilson, the pioneer of oestrogen therapy (HRT) and author of *Feminine Forever*, in 1966, wrote about the menopause in terms such as these: 'the women becomes a eunuch', 'no woman can be sure of escaping the horror of this living decay' and 'she is incapable of rationally perceiving her own situation'. He advocated oestrogen therapy from 'puberty to the grave' to alleviate 'emotional and physical decline'.

Attitudes to the menopause are not just about negative *attitudes to women* but also about *ageism*: older women are treated differently from older men. Again, think of the ways we are sometimes described – old hen, old witch or bag, silly old moo or cow, battle-axe, old biddy, or old dear. Neutral or affectionate terms, such as old codger or old boy, are kept for men; 'old woman' is reserved for an insult! Even the tag 'menopausal woman' is often used disparagingly, and it is scandalous that a normal stage of female development should be used as a term of abuse, or as a joke. Most of you will have heard a woman's behaviour being dismissed by, 'Oh, she's going through the change.' The idea that women become confused and irrational during the menopause is widespread. Recently, I have read this in a medical textbook, 'the assumption has been put forward that women's ability to work reduces to a quarter of normal by menopause' (Achte, 1970). If these are the myths offered as 'facts' in specialist books, it is little wonder that they have influenced popular opinion and media stereotypes. But have they influenced *you*? What do you think about the menopause?

It is very difficult to tap our basic attitudes and beliefs; examine your own feelings. For example, a colleague of mine who is normally aware of ageism and sexism, recently confessed to me that she became angry when someone began to talk about the menopause over dinner. She was approaching the menopause and admitted that she did not want to be reminded about it. Being aware of your 'gut reactions' can tell you a lot about your own prejudices. How comfortable do you feel about discussing the menopause?

I asked over 700 women aged between 45 and 65, what they thought most women experienced during the menopause. Here are some of their answers:

- Hot flushes, tingling, irrational swings in mood, vaginal dryness and loss of libido.
- Hot flushes, no periods
- I have no idea or expectations, hot flushes, I suppose.
- Generally stressful, anxiety, old age, loss of child-bearing ability, marital stress – you are less attractive

as a woman. Alteration of skin texture, facial hair due to hormone imbalance.

- Extra weight, lack of confidence, irritability
- Depression, lack of interest in appearance
- Irregular periods, flooding, depression, hot flushes
- Most of my friends have finished their periods and there doesn't seem to be any set pattern.
- Extreme tiredness, headaches, woolly-mindedness, loss of concentration, possibly a temporary loss of confidence in oneself
- I think most women experience hot flushes. Your breasts become saggy, and a general feeling of ageing.
- Gain in weight, loss of attractiveness, skin loses its bloom
- Depression due to thought of getting older, hot flushes, forgetfulness.

Most of the 700 believed that most women experience hot flushes, but almost two-thirds also believed that emotional changes occur, and about half thought that women suffer from physical problems. Remarks about the menopause were generally negative – only 2 per cent of the answers could be classified as positive.

In contrast, when they were asked about their own *personal expectations* of the menopause, their attitudes were definitely more optimistic. More women made positive statements about their future menopause, and fewer expected emotional or physical changes or hot flushes. For example, one woman said, 'I think that most women really dread the menopause because your body alters and you are never really the same afterwards. But I do believe that if you have an active life and have reasonable health, as I hope I have, then it need not be too bad.'

There is a common, probably beneficial, tendency in all of us to believe that while everyone else might suffer problems at a particular stage of life, it won't happen to me. *I'll be the lucky one!* But as we will see, these general, stereotyped beliefs do appear to *influence* our experience of the menopause.

As well as putting open questions to them, I asked women to either agree or disagree with ten specific statements. See what you think before you read on. They were taken from medical and popular literature about the menopause, and are listed in the box below.

Beliefs about the menopause. Do you agree?

1 The menopause is an experience that depends upon your attitude of mind.
2 The menopause is a disturbing thing that most women dread.
3 The menopause marks the beginning of old age.
4 It is good to be free from periods at the menopause.
5 After the menopause, women are more interested in sex than before.
6 The menopause is psychologically upsetting.
7 Women enjoy sexual relations less after the menopause.
8 The menopause brings problems with physical health.
9 Men are less interested in women after the menopause.
10 Women are pleased that they can no longer become pregnant after the menopause.

It is important to remember that for the majority of women interviewed the menopause meant relief from menstrual periods and freedom from the risk of pregnancy. Many felt that the menopause was to some extent dependent upon your attitude of mind, which suggests that a lot of women regard it as something that they can influence themselves, rather than it being purely determined by biological factors. However, for some women, the menopause was linked with particular stresses. For example, around 40 per cent saw it as a disturbing event bringing both physical problems and emotional distress and others also linked the menopause with the beginning of old age. Ideas about sex and the menopause were mixed: about a third thought that women's sexual feelings increase, while a similar proportion believed that sexual enjoyment decreases. Very few women, however, thought that men are less interested in women after the menopause.

A recent study of women living in Manitoba shows that Canadian women have the same mixed feelings.[1] The majority agreed that the menopause brought a sense of relief, but they also believed that postmenopausal women are more often depressed and irritable. However, comparing these recent findings with an earlier study of European women,[2] attitudes today do appear to be slightly *more positive* than they were twenty years ago.

In general younger women seem to have more negative attitudes about the menopause than older women. Women also tend to have more positive views about the menopause after their own menopause than they did before it.[3] So it seems that first-hand experience and understanding what actually happens during the menopause can lead to a more positive impression. There is clearly a need to reassure younger women about the menopause.

So there are reasons for optimism: less than half of us

expect physical and emotional problems and the majority of us welcome this stage of the reproductive cycle. But don't be complacent – your attitudes are still probably more negative than they need be!

WHERE DO THESE STEREOTYPES COME FROM?

Most of you will probably have seen articles about the menopause in magazines or newspapers, or heard comments about it on the radio or television. There has been a marked increase in newspaper, magazine and radio coverage in recent years – although this has come from extremely small beginnings. Most reports take a medical perspective – viewing the menopause as a syndrome of many different symptoms, and recommending oestrogen therapy as the best remedy. However oestrogen therapy is a controversial treatment and newspaper articles attract volumes of letters both for and against it.

> Rather than wait for the menopause to attack, it is now possible, with a simple test, to determine the degree of oestrogen deficiency and to take HRT to forestall any unpleasantness. Shusha Guppy, *Observer*, 18.3.84

> Osteoporosis. . . . it plagues women from adult on, and reaches crisis stage at the change of life. Anthea Gerrie, *Daily Mail*, 16.10.87

> The fact is that many women are suffering from a definite deficiency disorder, just like diabetes or those with underactive thyroids. Joan Jenkins, Women's Health Concern, *Daily Telegraph*, 31.1.89

Everyone comments on how rosy my skin is. I can nearly always tell if someone is taking HRT by the quality of their skin. Teresa Gorman, *Daily Telegraph*, 31.1.89

. . . It is most important that the women who are users or potential users of HRT are aware of the fact that there is continuing debate about the potential benefits and risks of the therapy. Kate Hunt, *Observer*, 24.7.87

It is not clear exactly how we arrive at our own expectations of the menopause. Our attitudes may be influenced by our mothers, aunts or grandmothers and perhaps by our feelings about menstruation. Then the views of our friends and colleagues may also be very important and we are unlikely to be immune from images of middle-aged women presented by the media, soaps, plays or advertisements. Contact with doctors is also an important source of information.

Doctors, nurses and women's attitudes to the menopause were compared in a recent study carried out in California.[4] The doctors were family doctors or gynaecologists, and the women were all either menopausal or postmenopausal. The doctors and nurses consistently saw the menopause as a more 'disease-like' event than the women. They believed that symptoms, such as hot flushes, dizziness, sleep problems, depression and headaches, occurred more frequently and more severely in menopausal women than the menopausal women themselves. The doctors also had a more favourable attitude to oestrogen therapy than the women.

In another study, American women's views about oestrogen therapy, their attitudes to the menopause and their personal expectations were explored.[5] The researchers found that women were very divided on the issue of oestrogen therapy. They did not expect changes in 'femininity' or sexuality but the majority did view it as a medical problem – that is, something that produces symptoms that can be cured by medical treatment. These women were influenced by the 'disease' view of the menopause. At the same time they were confused and unclear about whether they should pursue treatment.

WHY THESE MYTHS?

If a large section of the population is viewed as unstable, irrational, crippled, depressed or as a figure of fun, they can be dismissed as inferior and need not be taken seriously. Jokes and embarrassment are a way of distancing ourselves from the discomfort of this image.

Women's bodily processes – menstruation, pregnancy and breastfeeding – are still tinged with shame, distaste, embarrassment and fear. The menstrual taboo has existed for centuries. There is an almost universal fear of menstruation and a long-standing link between the womb and emotionality. Menstruating women were and sometimes are viewed as having evil and very destructive powers; in different places and at different times they have been cursed with the ability to damage crops if touched, to cause impotence in men if touched, to curdle milk, to cause premature ageing in men if they set eyes on menstrual blood, and to rust mirrors, tarnish brass and blunt razors.

As a result, in many cultures, women are or have been excluded from certain activities, isolated during menstruation, punished and treated as dirty and inferior. Much has been written about why men should view women in this way and about how this reflects a basic mistrust and envy that exists between the sexes.

Freud and other psychoanalysts, writing in the 1920s, believed that women suffer from penis envy. Freud thought that women believe that they once had a penis but that this had been lost or castrated and menstruation is a reminder of this loss. Men's fear of menstrual blood is explained by their own fear of castration. They are afraid it might happen to them too! Emotional distress in women, such as premenstrual tension and depression, was explained in terms of reactions to loss of the penis. Having children was the only major compensation for not having a penis, and being a mother and a wife was regarded as the natural and normal role for women.

At the menopause we might expect to be freed from the menstrual taboo and be treated with equal status. But no! According to Freud and others, at the menopause we return to feelings of grief and loss and penis envy, because our only compensation – being fertile and having children – has passed by. We are described as 'losing our sexuality and femininity', as becoming 'unladylike and intolerably garrulous', and 'expressing anger and not wanting to do domestic chores'.

These early psychoanalytic writers reinforced the view that women are really second class citizens. An alternative argument was developed by the female psychoanalysts, in particular Karen Horney and Melanie Klein. Horney talks about men's basic 'dread of women'. Instead of penis envy she describes a more fundamental male envy, the 'envy of pregnancy, childbirth and motherhood, as well as envy of breasts and of the act of suckling'.

Melanie Klein emphasises the importance of 'womb envy' and of the powerful role of the mother in early child development. She focuses particularly on the envy and wish to damage the mother on the part of both male and female infants.* So in order to protect themselves from such envy and a fear of 'the powerful mother' – in other words all women – the power relationship between the sexes had to change. Social stereotypes about menopausal women are seen as a continuation of general misogynist (or women-hating) attitudes. It would be comforting to know that these views are things of the past but sadly it seems that this is not the case. Recently several authors have drawn attention to the subtle and not-so-subtle way that 'fear and loathing of women by men is alive and well',[8] and how such attitudes towards women are reflected in our educational, religious and legal systems.[9]

It is not only men who hold such attitudes. Women too can be influenced by these negative images.

I am not suggesting that no changes occur during the menopause. Rather, the changes that do happen need not be feared or seen as crises or catastrophes. Menopausal women are *not* second class citizens; they are not inferior to men or to younger women. In helping to challenge these negative stereotypes, you are helping yourself.

---

*Much early psychoanalytic theory neglected the psychological development of women, however during the past twenty years female psychotherapists have been redressing the balance.[6,7]

3

The Menopause and Beyond – What Really Happens

Most women have fears about the menopause. Many expect it to bring a host of physical and emotional symptoms, including tiredness, irritability, insomnia, hot flushes, sexual problems, wrinkles, weight gain and brittle bones. But are these stereotypes of menopausal women accurate?

We now have the information to understand what really happens more clearly, thanks to four major studies which were set up in the 1980s in North America,[1,2] Norway[3] and South East England. (For details of my own study[4] see page 160.) These projects are unique because the same women were monitored before, throughout and then after the menopause. The results all demonstrate that the menopause is only one of a number of factors that might influence a woman's health and well-being during this stage of life.

Personal and social factors – your health and lifestyle before the menopause, your beliefs about it and whether you are exposed to undue stress – are also crucial in affecting your experience of the menopause. This explains why your menopause might be quite different from your friends.

HOT FLUSHES

Do All Women Have Them?

The number of women who have hot flushes is lower than medical textbooks would generally suggest. Rather than the frequently quoted high numbers of menopausal women, between half and two-thirds of the women asked in Norway and South East England had this symptom. So quite a few women have no flushes at all. And a fact that is usually overlooked is that about one in seven women, who are menstruating regularly, say that they sometimes have hot flushes *before* the menopause. So the increase in hot flushes at the menopause is perhaps not as dramatic as we previously believed.

Night sweats can occur with or without hot flushes, but they generally affect fewer women. Just over half of the postmenopausal women (when periods have ceased) and just under half of the perimenopausal women (when periods are irregular) had night sweats.

Hot flushes become less frequent with age. Of the older postmenopausal women (aged between 56 and 65) I asked, just under half were still having hot flushes and about a third night sweats. Usually they stop within a year or two, and some women have them only for a few weeks, but for others they can last ten years or more. Some of the older postmenopausal women with flushes had a later menopause.

It is the duration or chronicity of hot flushes that is debilitating for some women. For example, May, 54, had been having hot flushes for the past six years, 'Individually they are not too bad. I mean that if I knew that they would be gone next year I wouldn't mind. It's the uncertainty about the future that gets me down. After a long time they are tiring.'

For ways of coping with hot flushes, see page 121.

Are They Incapacitating?

Hot flushes are not necessarily a problem. To find out more, I asked fifty of the women who were having hot flushes to describe what it was like for them.

For most women hot flushes are not very frequent. About half of the women had one hot flush each day, but the rest had one a week or less.

Only one in ten women was distressed by her hot flushes. Those who found them upsetting also said that the symptoms interfered with their daily lives. For some, this was because of night sweats:

> Most nights I wake up with the sweats. I sit by the window to cool down before going back to bed. Some mornings I feel exhausted and it's an effort to get going to work.

> I wake up at night soaking wet, push off all the covers and then wake up a few hours later shivering.

For others the main problem was discomfort during the day:

> I must admit that I am embarrassed about them. I feel

How often do hot flushes occur?

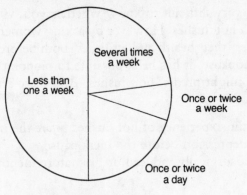

Are hot flushes distressing?

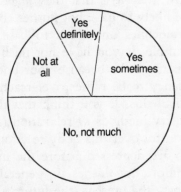

awkward and self-conscious, as if everyone's looking at me. I don't think I go red – I just *feel* so different. It is over in a few seconds though, and I just carry on afterwards and hope that no-one has noticed.

It's really uncomfortable. I feel hot and prickly all over and then I'm covered in perspiration when everyone else is not hot at all.

Can I Prevent Them?

It is very difficult to know whether you will suffer badly from hot flushes. However by asking women about themselves, their health and attitudes, both before and after the menopause, it has been possible to pinpoint a few factors that might predict hot flushes. And these are:

- the experience of hot flushes *before* the menopause
- depression before the menopause
- a surgically induced or premature menopause.

At the moment these are only tentative predictors and we do not know why it is that they *might* mean that a woman is more likely to have hot flushes. But you could use them as guidelines on which to base preventative action. For example, if you have hot flushes before the menopause, this might be because your bodily temperature has a tendency to be rather over-reactive. Blushing could be a sign of this. If you think that this applies to you, you could try methods of relaxation (see page 123) to gain more control over this body reaction.

Women who are depressed before the menopause do tend to report more hot flushes. In general people who are depressed view the present, the future and the world pessimistically; they tend to feel helpless and less in control of events around them. Also, when depressed, people are often more preoccupied with body changes, and from this perspective the menopause might be seen as yet another stressful ordeal to be endured. This state of mind could make the menopause into a more awesome event and so hot flushes could be more difficult to cope with. They might be the last straw when someone is only just about coping already.

Another, but not incompatible, explanation comes from recent studies which suggest that oestrogen levels are lowered when women are stressed or depressed.[5] A reduction in oestrogen levels then increases the likelihood of hot flushes. This seemed to be the case for Irene, who was taking oestrogen therapy (HRT) for hot flushes and who also had emotional problems, 'I am fine on the treatment for a while, but when the problems with my son get worse and I start to get depressed again, the hot flushes come back. It's strange, as if the extra worries use up the oestrogen.'

It is therefore advisable to seek help for emotional problems and find solutions, if you can, before the menopause. Talk to your GP about local counselling services; there are facilities for women with particular problems, some of which are listed on page 166.

The women I spoke to who were postmenopausal between 45 and 47, tended to have more hot flushes and to find them more distressing. Physical symptoms that occur before they are expected might well be more upsetting and they are less likely to seem natural. One woman, aged 45, felt very strongly about the timing of her menopause even though it is quite normal for it to occur at her age, 'Yes I have hot flushes. OK if I was 50, I wouldn't mind, but they constantly remind me that I'm *already* menopausal. None of my friends are. I just feel the odd one out and older as a result.'

If some women react like this to a menopause in their forties then the impact of an even earlier one is likely to be far more severe.

Surgical menopause also tends to result in a higher level

of hot flushes. This is probably because of the more rapid decrease in oestrogen. If you have a premature menopause, for either natural or surgical reasons, it is important that you seek information and support from others. The women I spoke to derived most benefit from regular group meetings, where they share their concerns and learn how to cope with problems as they arise. Turn to pages 82–83 in Chapter 4 for more about early menopause; for advice about coping turn to Chapter 7 and pages 163–4 for support groups.

While the rate of change in oestrogen levels is one factor determining whether or not you have bad hot flushes, your mood, your general health and your attitude will also play a part. What you can do is to try to improve your chances of passing smoothly through the menopause. For more about how to prepare for the menopause see Chapter 6. Remember that only a few women have troublesome hot flushes and these can be helped, see pages 121 and 136.

SEXUALITY

Satisfying sexual relationships *can* continue throughout and well beyond the menopause. This is clear from the recent studies of menopausal women, but it is a fact that contradicts traditional attitudes about this stage of life.

Women's sexuality is very difficult to assess. Vaginal dryness is not usually seen as a problem unless it causes discomfort during sexual activity. Similarly, measuring sexual arousal or interest presents a multitude of problems. Sexual interest or 'libido' is often gauged by the frequency of *intercourse* but of course this is misleading – many women enjoy sexual arousal by masturbating or mutual caressing.

Sexuality and Ageing

In the first major investigation of sexuality in the USA, Kinsey found that the frequency of intercourse and orgasm (between married couples) decreased with *age*.[6] However, there seemed to be no corresponding decline in women's solitary activities, such as masturbation, until well beyond the age of 60. Men are also less sexually active and experience more difficulties with intercourse as they get older. In fact, a recent investigation of men and women in Oxford clearly shows that men's sexual interest declines in their late forties and early fifties, but there is no parallel decrease in sexual interest in women of the same age.[7] In the largest study of female sexuality of all, Shere Hite illustrates the fact that for many older women sexual pleasure and desire continue and increase with age.[8]

Some people do find it hard to maintain or find a rewarding sexual relationship in later life. Boredom and habit are a common cause of this in long-term relationships. Women who embark on a new relationship in their forties and fifties tend to enjoy more lively and active sex lives than those approaching their thirtieth wedding anniversary. Another obvious explanation is the availability of sexual partners: women live longer than men and may find it difficult to meet a new partner, should they wish to.

Some women find that sex becomes less important to them as they get older and that other aspects of their relationships become more fulfilling. Others choose not to have sex at all. I have been asked by gynaecologists to see several menopausal women supposedly suffering from 'loss of libido'. As one women remarked:

I'm not really sure why he suggested that I come to see you. I did say to the doctor that we don't have sex very often – but we haven't for some years. We enjoy it when we do but the urgency has gone. He's happy with what's happening and so am I. It's not abnormal is it?

The answer is obviously no. We should not feel pressured to be sexually active if we do not wish to be.

Other women describe a new lease of life in their forties and fifties, and are ready to revitalise their sexual relationships:

After the boys left home I spent a lot of time thinking about myself and what I wanted to do. I imagined being on my death bed and looking back – what regrets might I have. One was that our sex life could be better. We're a bit lazy so I talked it over with Bill and things are now looking up. It is hard to change at this stage but it's worth it. The other resolution was to share the housework and shopping, and I'm still working on this one!

So *age* can affect sexual interest and activity – but not necessarily.

Sexuality and the Menopause

Does the menopause, with its hormonal upheavals, reduce sexual desire or enjoyment?

For the majority of women I asked, sexual interest had

not changed with the menopause. Nearly half actually said that they had lost interest in sexual activity *before* the menopause. This rises a little in women who are going through the menopause or who have passed through it. If you are one of these women there could be several reasons for your lessened sexual desire.

One might be vaginal dryness. Just under half of post-menopausal women say that dryness leads to discomfort during sexual intercourse, but it doesn't only affect post-menopausal women. A quarter of pre- and perimenopausal women also said it was a problem. Anxiety, anger, insufficient stimulation, tiredness, relationship problems and lack of communication can all reduce sexual arousal, and hence lubrication. Many women have experienced this situation at some time or other.

Lower levels of oestrogen can cause vaginal dryness, which is why it is more common in postmenopausal women. However, the other explanations are still very relevant, even after the menopause, and factors such as anxiety can make matters worse. Anne's periods stopped several years ago, when she came to talk to me about her sexual difficulties:

At first [after the menopause] we carried on as usual, having sex once or twice a week. I did notice my vagina being gradually drier but I'd use some KY jelly, which helped. The problem [not wanting to have sex] began when I had sex, really to please John; I don't do this very often but I was not in the mood and I was worried about a difficult class I had to teach the next day. John had been feeling low all week. The result was that we had sex and it was terribly painful – I cried out and he lost his erection. We both felt bad but we didn't really talk about it. Since then I feel tense when he tries to penetrate – now I suppose I expect it to be painful any time.

The vicious circle of pain/tension/lack of lubrication/ pain is quite common. It is easily broken by spending extra time in relaxation and foreplay so that you both build up your confidence before penetration. In any case penetration is not always necessary for enjoyable sexual relations.

Night sweats are another reason why you might be less inclined to have sex during the menopause:

When I'm getting the sweats at night, physical contact is definitely not on. I get so hot and sticky it wouldn't be very nice. At least we laugh about it! The sweats seem to come in bouts and they are gradually getting less frequent.

I have just felt so *tired* this year with the hot flushes and more responsibility at work. When I get home by the time we've eaten I just want to go to bed – to sleep.

Your health and the health of your partner (if you have one), or worrying about health generally, can also reduce sexual desire. Some illnesses, such as diabetes and pre-scribed drugs, such as some given for hypertension, can diminish male potency. Sex can be harder following a hysterectomy or cancer of the womb or cervix. Under-standably you may feel very vulnerable but, in your own time, there is no reason why your sex life cannot return to normal. Julie described what happened to her:

After the operation [hysterectomy] the thought of penetration made me feel uncomfortable: I really wasn't sure what I was like inside. Recently, when I went back for a check-up I wrote down all the things I wanted to know, and the doctor drew me a diagram of my vagina and cervix and reassured me that we could start having sex, since it is more than six weeks after the operation. We are beginning and are taking it slowly until I regain confidence.

Expectations and attitudes about sex and the menopause influence what we actually feel. For one woman the menopause provided an excuse to reduce her husband's sexual demands:

I've never been that keen on sex. I liked the affection but to be honest I could take it or leave it. I was quite relieved when, during the menopause, John just accepted that I said no more often. Perhaps I should be more honest.

Another woman had a very different experience:

I've always enjoyed sex and I was determined that all this doom and gloom about the menopause wasn't true. I'm now 51 and my periods have stopped. I have the odd hot flush but sex is still good, if not better, as I don't have to bother about periods any more.

Several factors were associated with a lowering of sexual interest in the women I asked. The main reasons were:

- being under stress
- having marital problems

- ill health
- having negative attitudes to the menopause
- having severe hot flushes or vaginal dryness.

If your interest in sex dwindles during the menopause, hormones are not necessarily the cause. Vaginal dryness, hot flushes and night sweats, tiredness and negative expectations can curb sexual feelings. It is quite understandable and normal for your sexual feelings to be sensitive to these changes too. The idea that hormones have a major impact on sexual desire is not supported by the results of recent studies: female sexual interest is not primarily determined by levels of oestrogen, leuteinising hormone (LH) or follicle stimulating hormone (FSH).[9,10,11] Testosterone, a hormone sometimes included in oestrogen therapy, is often thought to increase desire but there is no conclusive evidence that this treatment is helpful; instead counselling is more effective for sexual problems.[12] The only sexual symptom that is clearly linked to oestrogen levels is vaginal dryness, and this does not affect all postmenopausal women.

When I asked women about overall satisfaction or dissatisfaction with their sexual relationships there was an overwhelming statement of satisfaction both before, during and after the menopause. Eighty-one per cent of premenopausal women were satisfied compared with 84 per cent of postmenopausal women.

Couples do seem to make adjustments, just as they do during pregnancy and the postnatal period. The intimacy gained from *understanding* about menopausal changes can in fact be beneficial. Mary and Phil were 55 and 57 when they came for counselling. Mary had vaginal dryness and she was using KY jelly, but she had become anxious about sex. They had always been rather shy and inhibited about their sexual relationship, as Mary describes:

> Before we came here we didn't talk about sex. We love each other and enjoyed being close but we didn't know what each other liked and how we could please each other. Now we've spoken about it openly I feel more relaxed and this whole area of our life is more enjoyable and light-hearted.

INSOMNIA

> I lie in bed at night and all the day's worries go round and round my head. The more frustrated I get with myself, the harder it is to sleep.

> I realise that you need less sleep with age, so I deliberately go to bed a bit later when I'm really tired, then I sleep better. I also try to relax at some point during the day.

Sleep can be a problem at any time of life. If you are worried, depressed or very tense, poor sleep patterns can develop and they are difficult to shake off. It is true that you require less sleep with age. Some people have naps in the day because of sleeplessness but this only makes matters worse – save sleeping for the night time.

The menopause comes at a time when changes in your life resulting from age may be first noticed, so it is frequently blamed for problems which are in fact to do with ageing. Peri- and postmenopausal women generally

complain of more difficulties with sleep than premenopausal women, and disrupted sleep is likely to be exacer-
bated by night sweats and worries about the menopause.
Severe night sweats can certainly wake you up. When
oestrogen therapy is used to treat hot flushes, insomnia
becomes less of a problem too. But the treatment is not
so beneficial if you also suffer from persistent worries or
other emotional problems.

An important point to remember about sleep is that
there is a difference between having the odd night of
insomnia (or difficulty in getting off to sleep) and a recur-
ring pattern of waking early in the morning (about 2 or
4am) and not being able to go back to sleep. While the
former is common and can occur when you are tense or
feeling low, early morning waking can be a sign of more
severe depression.

If you think that depression is the cause of sleeplessness
for you, talk to your GP about the medical and psychological help that is available in your area. If not, then
exercise during the day and relaxation in the evening (see
page 123) should help, together with a good diet, avoiding
stimulants such as tea, coffee and alcohol. Some women
find that milk or camomile tea is calming at bedtime.
Above all, try not to be too worried about not sleeping –
most people can manage on less than they normally get.

URINARY FREQUENCY AND STRESS INCONTINENCE

Many women in their fifties onwards may find that they
need to rush to the toilet more frequently and have less
bladder control than they used to. Stress incontinence

means that a little urine is passed when you cough or laugh or are engaged in physical exercise. There was no real increase in women's reports of these symptoms at the menopause, instead they became gradually more common with age; just over one third of the women in their late forties and fifties said that they had noticed having to pass water more frequently than when they were younger.

While decreasing oestrogen levels can lead to reduced bladder control in some women, other factors are probably more important. These include weakened pelvic (or pubococcygeus) muscles caused by childbirth, general wear and tear, lack of exercise, obesity or chronic constipation. And urinary tract infections and diabetes can also lead to incontinence.

There are special exercises which strengthen your pelvic floor muscles and these can also be used to help prevent these symptoms (see page 124). If they become very persistent or troublesome your doctor may refer you to a urologist who might advise pessaries or surgical repair.

WEIGHT, SKIN AND HAIR

The thing that many women fear about the menopause is losing their looks. Several I have spoken to want to take oestrogen therapy in order to maintain or improve their appearance. But what are the facts?

Generally, the women in my study did not find that their weight increased during the menopause. Some women do put on weight in their forties and fifties, but with a good diet and regular exercise this need not happen (see Chapter 6).

There is an important difference between being overweight, in other words having excess body fat, and abdominal bloating caused by water retention. This is something that some women do experience at different phases of the menstrual cycle and during the perimenopause, but it will pass as your hormones settle down. You can help to reduce bloating by cutting down on salt and by eating foods that are natural diuretics – celery, parsley or grapes. Again exercise is likely to alleviate feelings of bloatedness.

Wrinkles and deterioration in the tone and moisture of the skin are often the first noticeable signs of ageing. With age, the skin usually becomes less elastic and may appear to be more translucent or thinner. Brown marks or age spots gradually become more common. One woman remarked:

In my fifties I did notice my skin becoming drier, more wrinkled and also itching in places. I used tons of moisturiser which helped but now I wish I'd taken more care in my thirties and forties.

The appearance of your skin during the menopause will be strongly influenced by your age, health and the way you have treated it during your life. Prolonged sun bathing and lack of creams and moisturisers can lead to dry skin and wrinkles.

Recent studies have pointed to a relationship between oestrogen and the amount of collagen in our skin. Collagen forms a bed of tightly packed fibres supporting the skin and it helps to maintain the skin's elasticity. There is some evidence that collagen and skin thickness decrease with reductions in oestrogen levels during and immediately after the menopause. So it is possible that the menopause could have a direct effect on the skin's appearance.

So is oestrogen therapy the answer? We tend to hear from people, especially politicians or film stars, who claim dramatic improvements in their skin after oestrogen therapy, rather than from women who notice no difference during the menopause. Women who use hormone therapy mainly to improve their looks, a reason that is not recommended by menopause experts, are likely to have spent time or money on skin care before the menopause. I believe that skin care and a healthy diet before and during the menopause are probably the most important factors for healthy skin in middle age.

Hair does not change significantly after the menopause, although it may become thinner with age. In addition, some women find that body hair, including pubic hair, becomes thinner in later life. Some doctors have pointed to the improvements of hair and skin in some women who are taking oestrogen, but there is no real evidence that hair changes are actually caused by the menopause. If severe hot flushes are alleviated by oestrogen treatment, so that you feel better and less tired, you may well look better.

Most women like to look and feel good, but should we really try to look 18 as we enter our fifties and sixties? Are men less attractive with a few wrinkles? Can't we create a positive image of older women that is attractive to us? We are surrounded by images of attractive young women and it's not difficult to conjure up a positive picture of a much older woman – even if this is an idealised, rosy grandmother image. But what are women in their forties and fifties supposed to look like? It is up to the next generation to lead the way; the choice is *yours*.

OTHER PHYSICAL SYMPTOMS

A few women describe physical symptoms or 'odd sensations' during the menopause – tingling feelings in arms and legs, itchiness, dizziness, headaches, funny turns, aches and pains, rapid temperature changes, fidgety legs and pressure and tension in the head and neck:

> I have been having hot flushes for a while. Usually they last only a few minutes but sometimes I feel dizzy with them and have to sit down for a few minutes. It does pass and it doesn't worry me so much now but it did when it first happened.

> When the menopause first started I felt very tired and aching all over. My strategy was not to fight it but to make myself rest when I needed to. It's a bit better now and I'm starting to exercise more. I'm getting my old energy back.

While some women do have palpitations and odd sensations associated with hot flushes, there is also a tendency for women and often doctors to attribute rather non-specific symptoms to the menopause. The results of the large-scale research studies carried out in the 1980s clearly show that minor physical symptoms are not necessarily more common during the menopause. Instead they tend to occur in clusters and can be associated with emotional or social problems, poor health and stress. Again, age itself can bring on general aches and pains, especially if you lead a sedentary lifestyle. Obviously if you suffer from a major illness during the menopause, hot flushes might well be a burden you can do without. But they are not a sign of poor health: they are quite normal.

If you do experience physical changes or symptoms *during the menopause*, remember:

- *Do not* automatically blame the menopause.
- Monitor your symptoms yourself. Keep a daily note of them. Find out if they are associated with other symptoms, such as hot flushes, or with what is currently happening in your life.
- Apart from hot flushes and vaginal dryness most symptoms have other causes. However, even these specific symptoms are influenced by your health and lifestyle.
- For most of you, your health and well-being before the menopause are likely to determine your experience of it. Only a few women experience severe disruptions to their lives because of hormonal changes.

HEALTH BEYOND THE MENOPAUSE

Two major health problems – osteoporosis and cardiovascular disease (strokes and heart attacks) – do become more common in women after the menopause. Various health risks increase as we age, and we begin to age in certain respects well before the menopause. It is only recently that doctors have begun to identify links between oestrogen supplies and osteoporosis and, to a lesser extent, cardiovascular disease. Hormone replacement therapy, which was initially prescribed for the relief of hot flushes, is now being advocated as a long-term preventative treatment for osteoporosis. One leading gynaecologist and osteoporosis specialist claims that, 'HRT is a major preventative treatment – it stops osteoporosis, relieves depression and reduces the risks of strokes and heart attacks.'

So once again the menopause, or in this case a post-menopausal condition, is being viewed as an oestrogen deficiency disease. What evidence is there to back up this claim?

Osteoporosis

If I drink milk or take calcium during the menopause, will it help prevent osteoporosis?

How will I know if I will get osteoporosis in the future?

Should I take hormones for osteoporosis just in case?

What Is It?

Osteoporosis, meaning literally 'porous bones', is a condition in which bone density reduces, thereby causing brittleness and the fractures that can result can then impair mobility and can even be fatal. There are several forms of osteoporosis but the most common type occurs in women after the menopause. We now know that this is related to lower levels of oestrogen in the body.

Bone mass gradually reduces with age in both sexes, but older women are more prone to this process and tend to fracture their wrists, legs and hips more easily when they fall. They can become smaller too, if the spine becomes curved. While increases in wrist and spine fractures occur in 50 and 60 year olds, hip fractures do not really become evident until the age of 70 plus.

Osteoporosis is on the increase. The number of women, and men, who fracture their hips has almost doubled since the 1950s. Some experts describe it as a health problem of major proportions and these are some typical statements to be found in medical literature on the subject:

One in four women over 60 years becomes affected by bone thinning.

As many as 5 to 10 million women in the US and perhaps one half to one million women in the UK are potentially at risk from fractures as a result of the skeletal destruction which occurs in the postmenopausal woman.

20,000 women die every year in the UK in what has become known as the silent epidemic.

The victims of such fractures occupy 40 per cent of orthopaedic beds in general hospitals and cost the National Health Service (in Britain) over £165 million a year.

Reliable statistics on osteoporosis are difficult to obtain since many sufferers do not go to the doctor. In fact many people are not aware that they have the condition until they break a bone. While it is estimated that one out of four women of 60 will have appreciable bone loss, the exact number of women who will go on to develop fractures is unknown.

What Causes It?
Throughout life the skeleton is in a constant state of growth, breakdown and repair. The balance between these three processes varies with age. After the age of 35, bone repair becomes less efficient, so that the body gets rid of more bone than it replaces. Bone loss in women increases

more rapidly for three to five years after the menopause. Then the rate slows down again. The areas that are most affected are the bones of the spine, wrists and hips, which become brittle and are therefore more easily broken.

The high incidence of hip fractures can be partly explained by the increased numbers of older women in the population. And there are clearly other factors, in addition to the decline of oestrogen levels, that might make women in particular prone to osteoporosis:

- Women tend to have smaller bones than men.
- Many women have sedentary lifestyles and do not take enough exercise and smoke.
- Women tend to be calcium deficient, probably because of slimming diets and a trend away from dairy products.

The use of calcium as a treatment for osteoporosis is controversial. Although some doctors claim that high calcium supplements help after the menopause, most experts now stress that it is the regular intake of calcium well *before* the menopause that is important in strengthening bones and preventing osteoporosis.

Doctors do not understand exactly how reduced supplies of oestrogen influence the development of osteoporosis. Oestrogen seems to help prevent bone loss indirectly through its interaction with another hormone called calcitonin. This means that calcium is retained, which is essential for building and maintaining your bones. So after the menopause you are likely to make less use of the calcium in your diet and even if you take in high amounts of calcium, your body is less able to process it.

Are You At Risk?
What every woman wants to know is whether she will
be at risk of developing osteoporosis and whether she can
find out about this beforehand. Several risk factors have
been identified:

- Skin Colour – The fairer the complexion the greater
  the risk.
- Racial Differences – It appears from recent studies that
  you are more likely to develop osteoporosis if you
  were born in or if your ancestors came from Britain,
  Northern Europe, Asia, China or Japan, and that you
  may be less at risk if you are of African or Mediter-
  ranean origin. Black women of African descent are
  less prone to osteoporosis than white women. This
  advantage is also thought to hold true for black
  women who have always lived in countries, such as
  Britain, that have less sunshine.
- Physical Stature – If you are small boned you are at
  greater risk because you have less bone mass.
- Age of Menopause – Premature menopause and surgically induced menopause lead to greater bone loss at
  an earlier age, unless oestrogen therapy is taken at the
  onset of the menopause.
- Family History of Osteoporosis – Osteoporosis runs
  in certain families, perhaps because of a genetic influence on bone loss or rate of loss. However, similarities
  in lifestyle and environmental factors may also be
  important.
- Illness or Drugs – Women who have suffered from
  rheumatoid arthritis, insulin dependent diabetes,
  Cushing's disease or thyroid problems, or who have

been prescribed corticosteroid drugs for problems such as asthma, are more at risk of osteoporosis.

- Low Weight in Relation to Height – This might be because oestrogen is converted from adrenal androgen which takes place in fat cells.
- Life-long Low Calcium Intake – This leads to reduced bone mass prior to the menopause.
- Sedentary Lifestyle – High activity results in increased bone mass. Regular exercise is important to build up bone mass and is also beneficial after the menopause.
- Cigarette Smoking – There is evidence that smokers have a reduced bone mass at the onset of the menopause.
- Excessive Alcohol Abuse and High Caffeine Intake – These can both have an adverse effect upon bone formation, although heavy drinkers tend to have a poor diet, which may be a crucial factor.

If you fall into one or more of these categories, you are not necessarily destined to have osteoporosis. What every woman can do is to use these guidelines to assess her personal level of risk and adjust her lifestyle accordingly. But anyone with early menopause, a strong family history of osteoporosis or who has had a high-risk illness or has taken high-risk medical treatment might be advised to weigh up the pros and cons of hormone replacement therapy against the chances of developing osteoporosis.

The measurement of bone mass has been an important development in recent years. X-ray measurements are not sufficiently sensitive to provide information about bone density although they do reveal fractures, but recent advances in bone-scanning techniques have made it much easier to measure bone mass during or before the menopause, and thus to predict the risk of osteoporosis.

However, if you are worried because you think that you are at risk, do enquire about local and regional facilities. In some parts of Britain, it is now possible to get a referral on the National Health Service to a specialist centre. Alternatively, if you can afford it, private clinics also offer these services. Experts anticipate that these methods will have greater clinical use in future and, hopefully, large-scale screening facilities will become available.

There are various choices: computerised axial tomography (CAT scans) can give a reading of bone density, mainly from pictures of the spine. This method is widely available but does not detect very early bone loss. It can be uncomfortable and relatively large doses of radiation are used.

Single photon absorptiometry measures bone loss in the forearms, hands, legs and feet. This procedure uses very low levels of radiation and women usually say that it is not uncomfortable.

Dual photon absorptiometry is a newer technique. Its big advantage is that it can examine the spine and hips – the areas that are most susceptible to osteoporosis. It is the best method of detecting osteoporosis in younger women, as well as being cheaper than a CAT scan. These latter two methods, being new, are not widely available and repeated assessments are necessary to find out the rate of bone loss.

Oestrogen therapy can slow down the rate of bone loss after the menopause, but bone that has already been lost cannot be replaced. Long-term treatment is usually recommended starting as early as possible after the menopause and for at least five to ten years afterwards, then bone loss is delayed for as long as the treatment lasts.

However, the role of HRT as a large-scale preventative treatment is uncertain. *Osteoporosis*, produced by the Royal College of Physicians in 1990, concludes that, 'Until further information is available on the balance of risks and benefits of HRT, both in terms of disease . . . as well as the type of preparation . . . it is unlikely to be accepted as a population strategy' (see page 169 of the publication).

In view of these misgivings and since there is no cure for osteoporosis, preparation and preventive measures prior to the menopause are strongly recommended. There is a lot you can do to reduce your risk of getting osteoporosis as described in Chapter 6.

Cardiovascular Disease

Cardiovascular disease causing heart attacks and strokes are the major cause of death in the developed world. Men are at much greater risk of dying of heart disease than premenopausal women, although after the menopause the risk for women increases at a much faster pace. Even in very old age, on average men still have a slightly higher mortality rate than women.[13]

Is the Menopause to Blame?

The bulk of the evidence in favour of the oestrogen theory, that oestrogen protects premenopausal women, comes from two sources. First, large-scale population studies show that the earlier the menopause (whether it is naturally premature or surgically induced) the higher the risk of heart disease. Second, the incidence of heart disease is generally lower in women who are taking oestrogens.

Several studies point to a reduced rate of heart disease in women using oestrogens. For example the leading experts in this area, Martin Vessey and Kathryn Hunt, working at Oxford University, studied 4000 women who were prescribed oestrogen. They found only half the number of heart disease related deaths compared with the national rates.[14]

But of five major studies carried out in the UK, USA and Sweden in the 1980s, four suggest that oestrogens are beneficial but one does not: the Swedish study reveals some detrimental effects to oestrogen users who suffer from more heart and artery disease, in particular strokes and heart attacks.[15] One problem with this type of study is that women selected for oestrogen therapy are already a healthier group because they are screened for risk factors, such as high blood pressure and diabetes, before starting treatment. Consequently the findings of the Swedish study are especially worrying.

There are two additional pieces of evidence which raise doubts about hormone replacement therapy. The contraceptive pill (with synthetic oestrogen and progestogen) is known to increase the risk of thrombosis (clotting in veins) and strokes, and when men are given oestrogens – for example as a treatment for cancer of the prostate – they are more at risk of heart disease. The position is complicated further when we look at how oestrogen might act to protect premenopausal women from heart disease. High amounts of cholesterol in the blood are potentially dangerous. But substances resembling fat (high density lipoproteins) work to reduce the level of cholesterol in the body. Oestrogen is thought to increase these lipoproteins and so indirectly it helps to break down cholesterol. But oestrogens also encourage another fat (triglycerides), which actually causes blood clots to rise in the blood.

Progestogens, which are now prescribed with oestrogens to reduce the risks of cancer of the womb, appear to have the opposite effect to oestrogens on the fats in the bloodstream. For example, it is possible that the addition of progestogens might eliminate whatever good effects oestrogen might have on your cardiovascular system.

So while the weight of recent evidence suggests that premature menopause is associated with an increased risk of heart disease and that oestrogens can reduce this risk, there are still considerable concerns about the overall effects of oestrogens. Reviewing the recent evidence, Martin Vessey and Kathryn Hunt conclude that:

> . . . more research is required. We believe, however, that definitive answers about the general balance of benefits and risks associated with hormone replacement therapy will not become available until major investment is made in large scale controlled clinical trials.[13]

Are You at Risk?

There are few doubts that the following risk factors are associated with cardiovascular disease:

- high blood pressure
- cigarette smoking
- high cholesterol
- obesity
- family history
- lack of exercise
- stress.

By the time you reach the menopause you will already have a 'risk profile' and will be able to estimate your risk of developing cardiovascular problems. You should therefore try to reduce some of these risk factors beforehand. While the number of deaths from heart disease has been falling in most countries during the past twenty years, the UK lags behind and still occupies the position at the top of the coronary death league.

So, by starting to take positive steps to reduce your risks of heart diseases before the menopause, you will not only be preparing for a healthier life beyond the menopause, but you will be increasing your chances of reaching menopausal age itself.

DEFICIENCY DISEASES?

It seems certain that there is indeed a link between oestrogen and the risks of developing osteoporosis and heart disease. But the effects of long-term oestrogen therapy are not yet fully known, and its effectiveness has not been conclusively demonstrated in the prevention of cardiovascular disease.

We do know that premenopausal preparation can go a long way to reduce a woman's overall chances of developing these diseases. Moreover, unless women act to improve their health in this way, the postmenopausal years are likely to be viewed increasingly as the age of deficiency diseases. We must now harness the enthusiasm and energy that have gone into improving women's health and fitness in recent years, and direct them towards these longer-term goals. By doing this we will not only help ourselves but we will also start to change this negative image of older women.

4

Menopause and Your Emotions

Women become insane during pregnancy, after parturition, during lactation; at the age when the catamenia (menses) first appear and when they disappear (the menopause). The sympathetic connection between the brain and uterus is plainly seen by the most casual observer.

G. Fielding Blandford, 1871
(President of the psychiatric section of the British Medical Association in 1894)

Unfortunately these myths are, to some extent, still around today. In 1989 a leading British gynaecologist advocated the use of oestrogen (HRT) for premenstrual tension, postnatal depression and 'menopausal depression'.

Joan, anticipating her menopause said, 'I'm dreading it. Women go a bit crazy don't they? My job is demanding enough, I do hope that the menopause won't affect me so much that I can't keep up with my work.'

WILL I GO MAD?

No. During the menopause you are at *no* greater risk of major mental illness (that is severe depression, manic depressive psychosis or schizophrenia) than you are during other stages of life. Studies of the numbers of women admitted to psychiatric hospitals or going to their family doctors with depression, and large psychiatric surveys, all come to the same conclusion: the menopause does not cause madness.

It is time to challenge fears based on folklore and prejudice. This took a long time for Ruth, who came to see me because she was worried about her mental and physical health. Her mother had suffered from recurrent depression and Ruth, an only child, spent many years at home with her parents, looking after her mother. She became increasingly resentful about her lack of freedom and this was coupled with guilt about her mother's unhappiness. She felt trapped. When she eventually began to take steps towards making a life for herself her mother's mood deteriorated and it was during this time that her mother became menopausal. The family began to attribute her worsening symptoms to the menopause and by doing this Ruth's guilt was to some extent alleviated. But the link between menopause and depression became strongly fixed in her own mind. Fifteen years later she described her own fears:

> I know I'm beginning the change of life. You know I do get mother's moods, and from time to time, I find myself saying the sorts of things she used to say. I just don't want to end up like her. I know she became so depressed during the change. I'm really worried. I know

I'm making myself worse worrying – but any ache or pain I have now I interpret as a sign of mental illness.

In time she began to disentangle her feelings from the menopause. She was able to talk more directly about, and free herself from, her resentment, guilt and sadness.

WILL I GET DEPRESSED?

Depression seems to be a predominantly female problem. Women are twice as likely to be depressed as men. This is true of most countries with the exception of some developing nations such as India, Iraq, New Guinea and Zimbabwe, where the ratio is reversed. It is important to

---

WHAT IS DEPRESSION?

Severe depression	*Normal moods*
If, most of the time, you:	If sometimes you:
– feel profoundly sad and empty	– feel irritable
– feel that life is not worth living	– feel fed up
– have no appetite	– can't be
– wake early in the morning and sleep badly	bothered to do things
– have no energy or motivation	– feel tense and anxious
– feel guilty and blame yourself for everything	– feel sad and miserable
– derive no enjoyment from the things you used to do	– feel resentful and envious
	– feel angry

remember that this sex difference in depression is *not* greater during the menopausal years. If anything it seems to be younger women, women of child-bearing age, who suffer most.

Why should this sex difference exist? For centuries female depression has been put down to hormonal upheavals occurring during the menstrual cycle, the post-natal period and the menopause. However, the bulk of research in the past twenty years points instead to social and domestic factors – the stresses of work and children, lack of social support and chronic housing and financial difficulties.

The years immediately before, during and after the menopause can bring relief from some of these pressures, as well as raising new challenges.

Until the 1980s research into mood and the menopause was on the whole inconclusive. However, evidence is accumulating, from European and North American studies, that points to the conclusion that, while hot flushes do increase during the menopause, emotional symptoms *do not*. In Britain most of the women I asked were no more anxious, tense or depressed during the menopause than before. But some women, about one in ten, did feel low during or just after the onset of the menopause. Most were not severely depressed but their normal feelings of irritability, low self-esteem and not really enjoying things, were accentuated.

The women who described these feelings during the menopause tended to be those who were depressed before their periods ceased, who had negative beliefs about the menopause (that it brings physical and emotional symptoms) or who were not working outside the home.

If you are depressed you might be more apprehensive

about the menopause than women who feel great or comfortable with themselves. Women with low self-esteem tend to be more influenced by the negative image of the menopause because it confirms their own views about themselves. Again the message is seek help before-hand if you can.

The negative stereotypes about the menopause which exist in most western societies, do lead to suffering and distress. Who wouldn't feel irritated and without any self-esteem if she believed that her body and emotions were about to let her down profoundly? Some women who are anxious before the menopause feel relief when their fears and expectations are not fulfilled, but often negative atti-tudes lead to the symptoms that were feared in the first place – depression and anxiety about being menopausal. It is, in fact, middle-class women who are more likely to have such attitudes about the menopause. Perhaps they have greater exposure to, or belief in, the current medical literature, but we cannot know for certain. It is therefore vital that we help each other to develop realistic and more positive expectations about the menopause.

Working outside the home before the menopause seems to protect some women against depression. This tends to be the case when the work offers its own rewards, if it represents an escape from domestic stress, or if colleagues at work are friendly and supportive. But in some cases the menopause, with hot flushes and night sweats, can feel like an additional stress in an already very stressful life. This was the case for Pippa, 48, who had her last period six months ago:

I have a demanding job with many conflicting demands, and I have to organise my children [aged 9 and 12] to do their homework, et cetera. We also try to make some time for a social life. Before the menopause this was rather like a juggling act, but now, with the hormonal changes, it has all become more of a struggle. The hot flushes make me tired and my body seems to be telling me to slow down.

Women do often need permission to do exactly that. It can help to delegate some areas of work and take the pressure off for a while if your body needs it. Pippa did manage to do this although it was difficult at the time. Looking back she regards it as a helpful exercise for the whole family, because various jobs and responsibilities had to be shared.

Sandra works full-time as a catering manager and has lived on her own since she and her husband divorced two years ago. She has had hot flushes and irregular periods for the past year:

My menopause has affected me in a very general way. I can cope with the hot flushes although they do get on my nerves at times. The real problem is feeling more tense and irritable – not all the time, it comes in waves. It is the same sort of feeling as the PMT I used to have but now it's more frequent. As a result ordinary things are a bit harder to cope with.

Sandra's mood swings did appear to be partly due to hormonal fluctuations, although it is difficult to know for sure. One way to try to find out is to keep a record of your mood changes to see whether they follow a cyclical pattern (like the menstrual cycle). If so, it can be useful to concentrate on dealing with difficulties at other times of the month and relaxing more during the times when you feel vulnerable. For relaxation instructions see page 123. However, remember that these feelings should diminish as you pass through the menopause and your hormones restabilise.

One of the major problems for women during this lifestage, if they do feel low, is knowing *why*. I have been given repeated examples of depressed women visiting their doctor and being told, 'it's just your age, you've got to live with it', or, 'you're menopausal, that must be the reason. Have you thought of taking oestrogen therapy?' It is too easy to put all the blame on to the menopause; lives are complex, and there are many reasons why a woman might feel low.

It can be very helpful to talk over your problems with someone in order to work out why you are depressed. Counselling services are available in most areas (see page 166). Rather than necessarily needing long-term therapy, many women benefit from a couple of in-depth discussions to pinpoint the main causes of their distress.

OESTROGEN AND DEPRESSION

Although this is an area of controversy, low oestrogen does not appear to be a major cause of depression in menopausal women. Oestrogen levels in the blood are *not* lower in menopausal women who are depressed.[1,2] Similarly, studies of oestrogen and mood during regular menstrual cycles do not support the hormonal explanation of depression in women.

However, oestrogen does appear to have a small but specific effect on the central nervous system. There is some evidence that oestrogen activates the system, producing an energising or uplifting effect for some women. The beneficial or 'mental tonic' effect of oestrogen on women's moods and general sense of well-being is described by supporters of oestrogen therapy.[3] Women taking oestrogen therapy sometimes claim an improvement in their mood which is fairly non-specific. This is partly due to relief from hot flushes and night sweats, and partly due to the 'placebo' effect of undergoing a treatment with repeated interviews and hospital appointments.

While we cannot rule out the possibility that oestrogen might have a kind of anti-depressant effect, particularly if taken in high doses, there is not much evidence to support this view. It is important to remember that, even if this beneficial effect can be proved, it would be wrong to assume that depression in menopausal women is therefore caused by oestrogen deficiency. Anyone, whatever their age, might well feel differently if they are given high doses of oestrogens. (As described in the previous chapter, there is some evidence that stress itself may lead to lowered oestrogen levels and hence more hot flushes. A vicious circle can then develop – stress causes more symptoms which in turn become more difficult to cope with.)

If the personal and social causes of depression in a woman are ignored, or wrongly attributed to the menopause, then oestrogen therapy does not make these problems go away.

To have a biological or physical reason for feeling low can sometimes be reassuring and perhaps eliminate the need to think about your own personal problems any further. But in the long term this is not a good strategy. Yvonne firmly believed that her symptoms of anxiety and depression were part of the menopause. Her life had been made miserable for many years by marital problems but rather than face the very difficult task of dealing with the problems, she chose to blame a safer, physical cause:

> My main problem now is the menopause. If I didn't feel so emotional and tense things would be better at home. Dave [her husband] agrees that my problems are hormonal. In fact I'm able to talk about how I feel, and he's a bit more sympathetic now.

While this explanation might make life easier in the short term, Yvonne was really blaming herself or her hormones for the atmosphere at home. After several meetings with the couple they began to voice their anxieties about the relationship and this, rather than the menopause, became the new focus of their discussion – with promising results.

IS MID-LIFE STRESSFUL?

Phrases like 'change of life' or 'mid-life crisis' conjure up the image of a stressed and troubled woman in her forties or fifties. Middle age can be marked by all sorts of problems:

- unfulfilling work or retirement
- bereavements – particularly of parents or partner
- coming to terms with age
- marital and sexual dissatisfaction
- children leaving home
- ill-health

Clearly these factors have nothing to do with the menopause as such, but if they occur at the same time the real reasons for any distress can be easily overlooked. The menopause can be blamed once again!

The 'Empty Nest' Syndrome

This phrase describes a woman who identifies strongly with mothering and the traditional female roles and who finds little meaning in life when her children have grown-up. The evidence supporting this 'syndrome' comes mainly from descriptions of women who have sought medical help. However, in studies of ordinary women who were followed through this transition, the emptying of the nest is more often seen as a relief than a crisis! Some need for readjustment and change definitely exists but most women see this as a challenge and describe increases in their activities and morale during the changes.

Women whose children have left home are generally more satisfied with life. There does seem to be a relationship between higher rates of depression and the years that children, particularly young children, are at home – probably because of the demands on mothers, and frequent difficulties in managing to combine work and childcare. Of the women I spoke to, those who had a son or daughter still at home (about 60 per cent) when they were in their mid-forties to mid-fifties, suffered from *more* physical symptoms, such as headaches and tiredness, than the women who had 'emptied their nests'.

Women often have difficulty in admitting to themselves that, as much as they love their children, they have been doing the caring for long enough. Jane, 53, lives with her husband and two adult sons. One left home but returned when his marriage broke up. She inherited some money and they used this to build a house extension, but this did not work out well and actually produced more stress. Jane works part-time but spent many hours waiting on her sons – making their sandwiches, ironing their shirts – and found that she had little private time with her husband:

> Yes I do resent ironing their shirts. My husband and I never have any privacy. They are always in the sitting room with their girlfriends. . . . I wish they were more independent.

Her wish to recreate the old mother-son relationships at home conflicted with her need for time with her husband and their plans for their own future. As a result she felt immobilised with panic and depression. However, she soon began to admit her resentments and put her own feelings and her marriage first – with benefits to all concerned.

Bereavement

Many women experience their first main loss during their forties and fifties, be it a partner, friend, parent, grandparent, aunt or uncle. Death, like the menopause, is another major taboo and people often find grief very difficult to deal with, either in themselves or in others. But grief is normal and adaptive.

There are factors that can serve to cushion the impact of grief. For example, having supportive friends or family – someone to confide in – clearly helps people to adjust. Working outside the home can also help, but obviously

GRIEF IS NORMAL

Phases of grief

Numbness – usually lasts 2–3 days and temporarily protects the person from the full impact of the loss. At this stage people often need a lot of support and help with even the simplest decisions.

Despair – includes the painful feelings of anguish and distress. As well as sadness, it is quite normal to feel angry (with yourself, others or the deceased) and guilty or regretful. People often feel physically ill, with a hollow feeling in the stomach, breathlessness and lack of energy. Grief can similarly affect one's thinking. You can forget the person has died or see the lost person. Dreams of the deceased are very common. Sleep and appetite disturbances can also occur, as does a tendency to withdraw socially. Some people seek out reminders of the person, such as places or objects, while others actively avoid them.

Recovery – means that gradually the loss is being accepted and life is pulled back together with changes to accommodate the loss. At this stage (and the time taken is very variable depending on the closeness of the relationship) it becomes easier to think about the deceased without the painful wrenching quality that was experienced earlier.

Bereavement is a normal long-term process – don't deny or rush your feelings. Find someone to talk to and if possible reduce other pressures and demands since grieving uses a lot of energy. For bereavement counselling services see page 166.

the nature of that work will determine whether work offers a relief from stress or whether it adds its own pressures. But it is important not to rush back to work too soon and employers should recognise the need to grieve. The process can take some time – and that can mean months or years – depending on the relationship with the deceased.

Women who have suffered an early loss of a parent or brother or sister in childhood or the loss of their own baby or child, may be more sensitive to later losses. If the earlier death was not spoken about or grieved about enough, then the old feelings can be triggered and re-emerge in later life. New grief commonly combines with previous unfinished sadness, guilt and anger. Vicky, 49, lost her mother three years ago. Their relationship had been good and she felt that, following a long illness, it was really the best thing that her mother died when she did. But her father had committed suicide when she was 9 and the family had not discussed the event afterwards, and the force of her anger and guilt now pervaded her life. The experience of her recent grief opened the doors to her deeper, unspoken feelings. She resented her mother for not talking about her father:

If only I knew why. All these years I have blamed myself, and my relationships with men were affected. Although at the time I did not make the connection I must have really lost trust in men.

In time she gradually rebuilt an image of her father and began to free herself of some of the guilt and anger.

Now that attitudes have changed to some extent and there are more facilities for bereavement counselling – do seek help. There is always someone to talk to. You might find it hard to take the initial step, just as Barbara did. Having held her feelings about the loss of her father back for two years, she said, 'I can't cry. If I do, or if I talk about him, my feelings are so strong I'm scared I'll lose control or explode or go mad.'

She gradually overcame this fear, by talking about herself and her father with me at her own pace, and then she was able to talk about him with others at home. In time she learnt to accept her mixed feelings towards him.

For some women the menopause and loss of parents can bring home the fact that death comes to us all. This awareness can help us to appreciate the present and plan for the future if it is positively channelled.

IS THE MENOPAUSE A STRESSFUL TIME?

Roughly half of the 700 women I asked said that they had recently been under stress. But overall there were no differences between women at different stages of the menopause: stress does not increase or necessarily coincide with the menopause. I also asked them to describe what was stressful. Their sources of stress were quite diverse. The largest category included general family problems, such as a partner's ill-health, or arguments between particular members of the family. Several women were stressed by more than one problem. Irene, for example, found moving house, together with her husband's illness, difficult to deal with.

We all have a threshold of coping above which we become stressed. Don't be ashamed if your life circumstances push you to this level at times: accept help from others, learn to delegate, say no, and try to solve one problem at a time.

Over two-thirds of the women I spoke to were employed, either full-time or part-time. While many found their jobs stimulating, work often presented various problems. Many women were stressed at work, some were bothered by arguments with a particular person or felt undervalued. Unemployment was also mentioned as a source of stress.

I have a very demanding job as a school secretary. *Jane*

Being one of the few women at management level is exhilerating, but the politics and power games that go on take too much of my time and energy. *Amy*

Starting a new job earlier this year. *Tuohy*

Pressure in very demanding job and breakdown of a relationship. *Margaret*

No job, and I've broken up with my boyfriend. *Diane*

Changed job. *Minnie*

Under-staffing where I work as a nurse. *Ruby*

Work was mentioned as a problem less frequently by older postmenopausal women, probably because many had retired. But the number of women who had been recently bereaved increased slightly in the postmenopausal age-band. Most of them had lost a parent but one or two women had lost partners. Some were especially unlucky, like Elizabeth, 57, who lost both parents within three years, and her brother also had a stroke, 'I became terribly run down, and it was as if for several months I just existed.

I still miss them both dearly. If I have learnt anything, it is to appreciate people and what I have now.'

Children are often a source of problems, particularly for younger premenopausal woman. Conflict and worry about teenagers is a recurrent theme.

I have great difficulties with one of my daughters who is at university. She doesn't keep in touch and she expects money, et cetera, without giving anything herself. *Mary*, 45

I am concerned about my own poor health [recurrent pains and sleeplessness] and looking after my severely mentally-handicapped son, aged 22. *Pam*, 47

Not surprisingly, concerns about parents increased for the postmenopausal women. Women were worried about their parents' health, their ability to look after themselves and, for many, the practical strain of caring for sick relatives took its toll.

The menopause did *not* necessarily coincide with more problems in relationships, divorces or separations. But some women found relationships a considerable source of stress. Sue, 41, was unemployed but looking for work, 'I feel very lonely since I broke up with my boyfriend.'

Daphne, 53, was divorced last year, 'I dealt with the divorce well, and in many ways it was a relief. I began a relationship with a good friend a few months ago but it didn't work out, so I'm feeling a bit low at the moment. I'm going to concentrate on developing myself for a while. I want to learn to drive.'

Other general stresses included moving house, retirement, ill health, homesickness (one family had moved to

England from New Zealand) and many more, but very few women mentioned the menopause as a source of stress. Mid-life brings varied stresses and challenges for women, depending upon their lifestyle, but these are separate from the menopause and they usually have personal and social, rather than biological, causes.

But What About Fertility?

Most women will have made decisions about whether to have children or another child before the onset of the menopause and those last decisions are usually made in our early forties. By the time women in Britain are 35, more than half of them will have been sterilised and for the majority of women I spoke to infertility, or end of the reproductive phase of life, was not an issue. They were more concerned about the impact of the menopause upon their looks and their emotional and physical health. But for some the menopause may provide a reminder – perhaps tinged with sadness and regret – of past decisions or accidents.

In many ways we have had more choices than women of previous generations, for whom numerous pregnancies were mostly inevitable and arduous. Today many women are choosing not to have children. But exercising control and having choice can be very hard. Practical and biological accidents do happen. Your feelings may change at a later life stage and *all* choices naturally bring mixed feelings. Even if, for example, you decided on one child, you might emotionally feel a sense of regret or curiosity about what another may have been like and this is quite natural. It is a time *not* to feel guilty about your choices and to respect each other's decisions.

But some women, for whom the menopause comes too early, do not have the choice. Premature menopause, especially for younger women who have not even contemplated children, can be quite traumatic. They often feel cheated, as Pam did:

> I'm 32. I shouldn't be menopausal. I did intend to have children in the next few years but now what? I do feel resentful but it's gradually getting a bit easier.

When the choice of whether or not to have a child is taken away a common initial reaction is to want a child, even for those who did not previously plan to have one. These women often feel angry because their options are being limited, and there is frequently no one to blame. Women who are told they are infertile are in a similar position, but infertility is usually preceded by a process of investigation. For those women at least there is time to think about the options if treatments do not work.

The emotional issues raised by premature menopause vary depending upon a woman's age and lifestyle. For younger women in their teens and twenties, who do not have a regular partner, concerns are often about feeling different or abnormal. They have to come to terms with the fact that they are not menstruating, and how or whether to tell other people. One woman, Joanne, felt ashamed and guilty about being menopausal. She was concerned that she should not deceive a new boyfriend, and she discussed the impulse she had to tell potential boyfriends straight away. She found, however, that the particular person that she made friends with and eventually began to trust, accepted the situation more easily than she expected. For Joanne the menopause meant that she was more cautious in her relationships with men and needed to be reassured that she could trust them with her 'problem'.

Women who become menopausal in their twenties and thirties are mostly worried about the effects of the menopause upon their looks and physical health. They think that they will rapidly age. As one woman put it, 'I will be a young person in an old body.' She was wrong in fact. By meeting together these women could reassure each other, the younger women could see that life could be enjoyable for the older ones. They were faced with living evidence that contradicted their ideas about the menopause and ageing and decline.

For those women who badly want children, in-vitro fertilisation (test-tube baby technique) is now possible using an egg that has been donated by another woman. These methods can be emotionally harrowing and are, on average, only about 10–20 per cent successful. If you decide that this is the right decision for you, enquire about facilities in your health area. Unfortunately, only a few hospitals offer such services free on the NHS, and many women have to travel to South East England.

If we can begin to discuss the menopause more openly, then women who have an early menopause might not feel so unprepared. If you find that this happens to you, through natural or surgical means, there is help at hand. (See Chapters 7 and 8 for discussion of hormone treatment replacement and alternative therapies.)

It is important to remember that, contrary to popular belief, depression is *not* an inevitable part of the menopause. By challenging the idea of 'menopausal depression' and the traditional myths about 'menopausal madness', you can reassure other women and help to paint a more realistic picture of the menopause for everyone.

But if you do feel low, it does make sense to look to your relationships, to stresses and your lifestyle for the most likely causes. Take time to try to find out exactly why you feel like you do, and rather than deny your need for help and support, talk to someone – a friend, a colleague or a relative – or seek professional help if necessary. If there is a menopause group in your area you will probably meet women with similar concerns (see page 127). Put yourself *first* for a change.

5

The Menopause, Across Time and Cultures

Does the culture and age we live in influence how we experience the menopause?

If we feel valued as older women, will we have fewer symptoms during the menopause?

Has the menopause always been viewed as a crisis or a deficiency disease?

A brief journey into the past, and across cultures, brings us face to face with evidence pointing to the relative nature of the menopause and the importance of the *social* meaning of this life-stage. The menopause has not always been regarded as a disease, and if the circumstances are right then women can certainly look forward to this time of life.

A CULTURAL PERSPECTIVE

The menopause is often described as a western culture-bound 'syndrome' which affects mainly white women of

European origin. Most European and North American societies are now multi-cultural and racially mixed but unfortunately little is known about the menopause in non-western cultures, or in the various ethnic or social groups within western societies. But all the evidence that has been collected by anthropologists and social scientists suggests that the way we respond to the menopause is indeed conditioned by society's values, especially the esteem – or lack of it – in which older women are held, and the roles offered to them in that society. The key factors which determine the status of menopausal women are:

● Is age valued over youth?
● Is there a lifting of menstrual taboos?
● Is there a traditional and valued grandmother or mother-in-law role?
● Is reproduction highly regarded?
● Is there an extended family system?
● Is beauty or sexuality central to women's image?

A woman's status is often reversed after the menopause. For example, in societies with rigid menstrual taboos women enjoy greater freedom after the menopause. The anthropologist Margaret Mead discovered that both pre-pubertal girls and postmenopausal women in Bali had the same privileges as men. Similarly, the Lugubara women of Uganda become 'Big Women' after the menopause. They achieve social equality with men and may exercise considerable authority within the family.

Male and female behaviour in Islamic societies is clearly defined by taboos and social sanctions, which through western eyes often seem to discriminate against women.

After the menopause however, women can be unveiled, released from seclusion, and can talk and drink with men.

One of the first detailed cross-cultural studies was carried out by the American anthropologist Marsha Flint, who talked to women of the Rajput caste in northern India about the menopause.[1] The menopause, she found, is accompanied by a marked change in status: Rajput women who no longer menstruate can emerge from purdah and enter public life. They are free to visit other households and can join male gatherings to drink, joke and talk. Not surprisingly, the women look forward to this positive change, and when asked about their menopause they have *no* symptoms.

In some cultures, the menopause is not a particularly important event. Japanese women regard the general process of ageing as a more personally-relevant issue. They voice fears about 'how they will get by, living by themselves with husbands whom they may never have come to know very well, given the organisation of contemporary Japanese life'.[2] It is interesting that these fears, and the very real distress apparently experienced by some Japanese women, have not become health problems. They have not become medicalised or associated with the menopause: Japanese women report far fewer hot flushes than North American women.

The menopause does not always benefit women – Gisu women in Africa are known to have a higher suicide rate at the menopause than at other times. But these women are rejected both by their husbands and their own families when they are past child-bearing age, as they are no longer seen as assets to either group.

The widely differing experiences of women are clearly demonstrated in one of the most comprehensive studies of the menopause ever undertaken. Yewoubdar Beyenne, of the University of California, studied how Mayan Indian women in Mexico experienced the menopause compared with women living on a Greek island.[3] It is worth going into some detail here as these women's lives give a flavour of the numerous factors that can influence our experience of the menopause. Both groups of women live in villages relying upon subsistence farming. Both societies have menstrual taboos, and the women have broadly similar social roles – but their experience of the menopause differs radically.

In Mayan society being a good mother, housekeeper and hard worker is valued. Power and respect increase with old age. The mother-in-law in both the Greek and Mayan cultures occupies the most authoritative position as head of the extended family households of her married sons.

When menstruating, Mayan women are believed to carry an evil wind and if they visit a new-born baby the umbilical cord will start to bleed and the baby will die. Menstruation is thought of as the discharge of 'dirty blood that needs to be changed each month'. Fertility is highly valued, although pregnancy is an especially stressful and potentially dangerous time for them. The women marry early and continue to have children until the menopause. Sterility is legitimate grounds for divorce.

Similar menstrual taboos apply to the Greek women. A menstruating woman is not allowed to go to church because she is unclean; she must avoid contact with the family's wine (or it will turn to vinegar), bread (because it will not rise) and cheese (in case it becomes contaminated). Menstruation is seen as a curse brought on by Eve's sin, and women must suffer as a result. However, the Greek women have fewer children, two on average, largely for economic reasons, such as shortages of food. Their principal worry regarding fertility is unwanted pregnancies.

The menopause is *not* a problem for Mayan women. *No hot flushes* are reported by these women – they do not even have a word for them. Mayan women welcome this stage of life, they are pleased to be free from taboos and restrictions, as well as from periods and pregnancy. Ironically they associate this time of life with being young and free and many postmenopausal women in the study said, 'I feel like a 6-year-old!'

The Greek women are also pleased to be free from menstrual taboos and the fear of unwanted pregnancies. *But* to them, the menopause means growing old, lack of energy and generally going downhill. Postmenopausal women must wear dark clothes, and these Greek women are generally anxious about becoming menopausal. The startling contrast to the Mayan women is that three-quarters of the Greek women report having hot flushes and many of them suffer headaches, irritability and insomnia during the menopause. The word *exapsi* is used for hot flushes, which they believe to be the result of retained blood boiling up in the body.

This study dramatically illustrates how women's perception and experience of the menopause can vary across cultures. Not only do Mayan and Greek women's emotional reactions differ, but so do the physical changes which are regarded as the major symptoms of the menopause. Factors such as diet, genetic differences and age at the menopause probably contribute in part to these differences. Mayan women reach the menopause much earlier, and they are less well nourished than the Greek women. We know that diet can influence hormone production but its precise effects on menopausal age or hot flushes are not clear. In neither society is osteoporosis a problem. The diet of both groups of women is high in calcium and they maintain a healthy level of physical activity throughout life.

I believe there are four lessons to be drawn from these cross-cultural comparisons:

- The experience of the menopause is not fixed.
- The menopause can be a positive experience.
- The menopause may be influenced by many social factors, such as attitudes to menstruation and fertility, the nature of family units and the roles available to older women.
- Compared to other cultures the menopause in western society is perceived as an unduly negative life-stage.

You can help others appreciate that the meaning of the menopause is largely determined by wider social values. Talk to other women. Learn about their traditions and experiences, and they can learn from you. You might be surprised, as I was when I ran a workshop on the menopause in South London. Women attended from various backgrounds and cultures, and each described a very different menopause. One woman from the Bahamas told me:

We don't complain about the menopause and we wouldn't take hormones. At home women are pleased to finish with having children and are happy to be grandmothers. My mother had sixteen children. She feels better now she has less hard work and more fun.

Another woman, whose family had lived in South London for decades, felt differently:

The worst thing for me is the hot flushes. They come on when I'm not expecting them and I get embarrassed. People round here don't talk about things like this. I wouldn't go to to the doctor. I just try and cool down without anyone noticing.

GOING BACK IN TIME

The earliest references to the menopause as a medical problem appear in the eighteenth century. A common fallacy is that, prior to this, so few women reached middle age that the menopause was never an issue. A substantial proportion of women has always reached the menopause. Women have had a life expectancy of fifty years for the past few centuries at least. This is particularly true of upper-class women, and of women since the eighteenth century when there was a great increase in life expectancy.

Another common view is that there was once an age when women enjoyed considerable power and status – the era of matriarchy. There is some historical evidence to show that women occupied an important position in some societies in the 4,000 years or so between the emergence of the first civilisations and the birth of the major religions. Female gods were worshipped and women were held responsible for the mysteries of reproduction, fertility and the growth of crops. An increasing emphasis on man's involvement in procreation, coupled with changes in patterns of agriculture, are factors which may have contributed to the decline of female deities and the emergence of social structures and belief systems which bolstered male supremacy. While there are some doubts as to the existence of *absolute* matriarchies, there are certainly indications that earlier societies were more egalitarian and as a result, it is likely that menopausal women enjoyed greater respect and status.

While there is no direct record of the menopause in medical writing before the eighteenth century, there is indirect evidence of the 'treatment' of the menopause well before this. The major theory about the menopause – held by women, scientists and doctors – dates back at least as far as Roman times. Menstrual discharge was regarded as poisonous. After the cessation of the menses, toxins previously excreted via menstruation were 'retained'. They then destroyed the body from within. I have come across women who today still have similar notions. One 76-year-old told me, '. . . it's this tension. *You* don't get it, because for you it's released every month. After the change the tension is with you all the time.'

Numerous treatments were used to ensure a continuation of menstrual flow in order to rid the body of 'peccant matter and morbid humour, sometimes acrimonious and malignant . . . whose retention never fails to be extremely injurious . . . to the constitution'. Initially healers used 'remedies' such as emmenagogues (agents which promote menstrual flow), applying leeches to the genitals or encouraging bleeding by cutting veins. In addition, the excretion of 'retained poisons' through the gut or skin was encouraged by purgatives, enemas and leeches, as well as by sweating and bathing.[4] These horrendous treatments were largely sought by upper-class women in classical Rome, Byzantium and as recently as in the affluent courts of post-Renaissance Europe until the eighteenth century. Women's status during these times depended upon appearance, sexuality and attractiveness and so despite enjoying greater social and sexual freedom, they feared the physical decline and the loss of sexual attractiveness after the menopause. As a result, they apparently actively sought treatment, even though it almost certainly will have caused them terrible problems.

Menopausal and climacteric complaints were first treated by doctors in eighteenth-century France.[4] Economic conditions in Europe improved with more efficient agricultural practices and an end to the recurrent plagues of earlier centuries. Life expectancy rose. Again it was the upper-class women who initially demanded help from doctors. Nevertheless the treatment of menopausal women did not really improve and the theory of retained poisons prevailed until the end of the century.

Around this time, the controversy over the menopause as a disease or natural state was beginning to be aired. In 1776, Fothergill, a British doctor, attributed menopausal complaints to the treatments being used, which were causing haemorrhages and infections, and he insisted that minimal treatment was necessary. His knowledge of the menopause came mainly from women of the very new industrial aristocracy, who were God-fearing fatalists and who wanted nature to take its course.

French doctors took for granted that peasant women were unaffected by the menopause, but not the sensitive and refined women of the upper classes, and France became the centre of menopause study. Several books and theses were written. Although physical problems, such as haemorrhage, were the focus of much attention, changes in *temperament* and *emotional symptoms* were added to the 'menopausal syndrome'. One of these early books was by Gardanne, who in 1816 was the first to use the term '*menespausie*', which he later shortened to menopause.

It was not until 1857 that a link was discovered between the functioning of the ovaries and the menopause, until this time, and for several decades afterwards, the menopause remained a French 'disease'.[4] The moral and religious ethics which dominated not only British Victorian society but also North American and to a large extent French and continental life meant that women who did not have children were stigmatised, and sexuality was in general suppressed. Symptoms of the menopause were often blamed on earlier sexual indiscretions, and the expression of sexual desire by menopausal women was considered ludicrous or tragic.

The industrial revolution led to a greater division of work roles between the sexes, especially for working-class women, and this created a doubling of pressures. They were required to continue to look after the home and children and also to work long hours in a factory or mill. We cannot know for sure, but in view of the general hardship and poor health of urban working people, it would not be surprising if the menopause was not often a major preoccupation among these women. In contrast, middle-class women remained at home.

As gynaecology began to flourish, many emotional as well as physical symptoms were regarded as being sexual or 'hysterical' in origin. Gynaecological surgery, including hysterectomy and clitoridectomy, was performed for insanity. Psychiatrists produced theories of female madness which were linked to the 'biological crises' of a woman's life cycle – puberty, pregnancy, childbirth and menopause – during which the mind would be weakened and symptoms of insanity might emerge.[5] In 1877 Krafft Ebbing wrote that the menopause could cause psychosis and personality changes such as irritability, discontent and quarrelsomeness. The diagnosis of 'involutional melancholia' – psychosis at the menopause – became widely used. Accounts of sexual changes also emerged, usually a loss of sexual interest but also increases or *'crises erotiques'*. Treatments suggested for these 'symptoms' of the menopause were so unpleasant that they must have deterred women from admitting any distress: doctors introduced ice into the vagina and applied leeches to the labia and cervix.

Bedrest was a common therapy for middle-class women who showed signs of discontent or who did not conform to their restricted domestic roles – a treatment which in turn led to increased isolation. Victorian women writers such as Florence Nightingale and Charlotte Brontë show quite clearly that it was the lack of meaningful work, hope or companionship that led to depression or breakdown among many women. And another strong belief in psychiatric circles of the time was that work, competition and activity would have grave consequences for women's mental state and reproductive capacity. Psychiatrist Henry Maudsley warned that intellectual pursuits for women would lead to 'a race of sexless beings'.

The menopause by the end of the nineteenth century had become a dustbin term, like hysteria, which could be used when women's distress was difficult to understand. In contrast, women doctors, such as Mary Putnam Jacobi and Elizabeth Garrett Anderson, vigorously refuted these ideas and from the 1870s onwards, the battle over the position of women in society, their civil rights, and their need for proper healthcare began to take real shape.

Psychoanalysis, a theory which developed out of the nineteenth century, promoted the idea of menopause as a *neurosis*. Again a pessimistic picture was painted, in which women mourned their loss of femininity and sexuality. As late as in the 1940s Helene Deutsch described it as a 'justified grief in the face of a declining world'.[6] Successful psychotherapy was difficult for women of menopausal age, she felt, since there was so little in the way of substitute gratification to offer them, 'for reality has actually become poor in prospects, and resignation without compensation is often the only solution'.

Menopause in the Twentieth Century

Two factors during the twentieth century have had a profound impact upon the treatment of menopausal women:

● the development of hormone replacement therapy
● the emergence of the women's movement

It was not until the 1920s that the main hormones produced by the ovaries were identified and the first injections of oestrogens were attempted in Germany and the USA in the 1930s. Stilboestrol, a synthetic oestrogen, was first manufactured in Britain in 1937. The 1940s and 1950s saw an increase in the use of hormone therapy, mainly for specific symptoms, such as hot flushes. What was at first a modest demand for treatment turned into a flood following publication in the USA of *Feminine Forever* by Robert Wilson in 1966. He listed twenty-six psychological and physical complaints that this 'youth pill' could avert – including hot flushes, osteoporosis, vaginal atrophy, sagging and shrinking breasts, wrinkles, absent-mindedness, irritability, frigidity, depression, alcoholism and even suicide. Women no longer had to resign themselves to their fate: 'total femininity' could be preserved. He argued that the treatment of women should begin in their thirties and continue until death.

Oestrogens were also recommended because of the advantages they could offer to the husbands of menopausal women by stabilising their wives' moods and improving sexual relations. Wilson gave an example of how he helped a distressed husband who had complained, 'She is driving me mad. She won't fix meals. She lets me get no sleep. She picks on me all the time and makes up lies about me. She hits the bottle all day. And we used to be happily married.' Following intensive oestrogen treatment, we are told that she resumed her wifely duties.

Feminine Forever was enthusiastically received in the USA and oestrogen sales rocketed. Within seven months of its publication 100,000 copies were sold and extracts appeared in many women's magazines. Premarin ('natural' oestrogen from the urine of mares) was the most widely used treatment and in 1975 it ranked as one of the five most frequently prescribed drugs in the USA.

Then, two independent investigations carried out in the USA linked oestrogen therapy with cancer of the womb (endometrial cancer) and oestrogen sales plummeted. Premarin slumped to twenty-fifth in the 1979 league table of most commonly prescribed drugs.

This cancer scare also served to focus American feminist attention on the menopause for the first time. There was concern too about the use of all sex hormones, including the contraceptive pill and DES (diethylstilboestrol). Women attacked the idea of the menopause as a 'deficiency disease' and asserted that the menopause was a natural event. They rejected oestrogen therapy as much for its social as its medical implications – for treating women as objects and reproductive agents and for using drugs as an insidious form of control.[7] For the first time women were encouraged to talk openly about their experiences and challenge attitudes towards the menopause and older women.[8,9] Alternative treatments for menopausal symptoms began to be explored.

Oestrogen sales have begun to recover since 1979 because the treatments have been refined, and oestrogens have been recommended for the prevention of osteoporosis, as well as hot flushes and other symptoms. Hormone therapy is now advocated in the USA and Europe more for its bone preserving benefits than its alleged rejuvenating properties.

But if we stop and think for a moment, women have been exposed to two quite polarised messages since the late 1960s:

- The menopause is a deficiency disease requiring oestrogen therapy, which if left untreated will impair the health and well-being of post menopausal women.
- The menopause is a natural event, which women can deal with on their own or with the support of other women, without medical intervention.

It is not surprising if you receive conflicting opinions and advice about the menopause and its treatment from friends, doctors, books and magazines. Don't be too concerned – just remember that your experiences and needs during this time are likely to be quite individual and might differ considerably from those of other women. Physical symptoms do occur during the menopause that may cause discomfort for some, and it is important that you do not deny the changes that might occur. But instead of using terms such as 'menopausal syndrome', with all its negative connotations, we should talk freely about specific symptoms, such as hot flushes. If we are frank and unashamed about ourselves we can go a long way forward, demolishing our own and society's prejudices about the menopause.

This brief journey across cultures and through history shows how rapidly and drastically attitudes towards the menopause can and have changed, particularly in the twentieth century. The key lesson for women is to remind ourselves about the *relative* nature of menopausal complaints and experience. We should also see how the treatment of women has served to some extent as a means of social control, legitimising sexist and ageist attitudes. The medical view of the menopause individualises problems and takes responsibility for change away from society. We have come a long way since leeches were routinely applied to our genitals, but the sad truth is that older women still occupy a low position in current western societies. It is up to us, and future generations, to produce positive images of older women who can be wise, who can have varied and important domestic, social and professional roles.

6

Prepare for the Menopause

Today most women take it for granted that they should prepare for childbirth. They know that they need to understand what happens during labour, and that this and a good diet and special exercises can give them more control over this event, in some cases without a real need for medical intervention. Similarly I believe that preparation for the menopause can yield enormous benefits to women. What is surprising is that we are not already applying this approach to the menopause, a process which every woman must go through. It is because many women dread the menopause and because their attitudes are still influenced by the myths surrounding it. As a result many premenopausal women prefer not to think about it. If we overcome this barrier we can begin to approach the menopause in a positive frame of mind. Preparation therefore involves challenging our expectations, being informed, having a healthy diet and taking the right kind of exercise.

CHALLENGING ATTITUDES

As I have discussed women who have unduly negative beliefs about the menopause are likely to have a worse experience of it. This is a 'risk factor' that you can change. Do you expect to deteriorate physically and suffer from emotional problems during the menopause? If so, ask yourself *why* you think like this.

The evidence from recent large-scale studies carried out in North America and Europe demonstrates that the menopause is *not* necessarily associated with general physical and emotional symptoms. Depression during this time is most commonly caused by social stresses or women's negative reactions to being menopausal. Physical symptoms can be due to ageing and illness and alleviated by changes in lifestyle. Most women's negative ideas about the menopause are unjustified.

For the women I have spoken to there are two common sources which feed these beliefs. One is their mother's experience of the menopause, the other is what they read in magazines, hear on the radio or gather from friends. Norma and Diana show how personal expectations about the menopause can be formed:

Well my mother prides herself that she sailed through the change unlike other members of the family, so I am keeping my fingers crossed that I will be as lucky as she was. *Norma*, 36

Most of my friends are in their early to mid-forties. We have all got demanding jobs and need to look good. Recently we have been noticing more articles about hormone replacement therapy in newspapers and magazines. We are all dreading the menopause – some of us think that when the time comes we will probably ask for HRT, but others are not so keen. *Diana, 42*

Although there is some evidence that the onset of the menopause can occur at a similar time for mothers and daughters, this need not necessarily be the case. For women whose mothers have had a premature menopause it makes sense to prepare earlier, but other factors are likely to influence when the menopause occurs, as well as how it is experienced. Your health and well-being before the menopause play an important part, and your mother might have had a poorer diet and a harder time generally earlier in her life. You are also in a better position to help yourself, and take preventative action.

We have seen how an entirely biological or medical view of the menopause, as currently advocated by some doctors, can reinforce the notion that the menopause is an illness. Doctors are likely to be biased, since they get their attitudes to the menopause from women who are having problems rather than those who are dealing with it well. You should also question what you read. The 'deficiency disease' view of menopausal women is to some extent a social creation and alternative positive images are equally plausible. The menopause can be another stage of a woman's life, a time to consider the past and make plans for the future, and a liberation from fertility.

It is important that you air your fears with others and discuss the validity of your beliefs before going on to develop a more positive perspective towards the menopause. Try talking about the menopause with family and friends. You might feel the urge to joke or make light of it or collude in a discussion of how awful it can be. But the more women talk about it openly the easier it will be. When I started working in this area I was conscious of wanting to say to others, 'Yes I'm very interested in the menopause but I'm not yet menopausal myself.' I didn't say this but the fact that I thought it at all reflected my presumptions about other people's reactions. Now it has become much easier. If you can begin a serious conversation about the menopause, women are generally very keen to continue the discussion. In the same way that many women feel confident enough to challenge sexist remarks by others, it is now time to draw attention to and to counter menopause myths.

When they are preparing for childbirth, women cannot wholly prevent the unexpected from occurring, and women approaching the menopause should not aim to have absolutely accurate expectations. For example, it is difficult to predict whether you will have frequent hot flushes or not. Julia, 49, has found her menopause difficult to deal with. She had always been fit and healthy and rarely visited the doctor:

First of all my periods became very irregular and I started to feel premenstrual and irritable. About six months later the hot flushes began. It wasn't that they were painful or anything, they were just so frequent. I felt hot and bothered most of the time, and they woke me up at night. I must admit that I've changed my attitude to people who have health problems. I used to think that they really brought it on themselves, or that most people made a lot of fuss about nothing. Now I'm much more understanding and realise that some things are just bad luck.

But what you can do is to know what to do if a particular problem like this arises. Having information and control over health decisions really does help. See pages 121 and 136 for ways of dealing with hot flushes.

REGULAR EXERCISE

Whatever your age you can improve your health and the quality of your life by exercise. But more often than not the thought of regular physical exertion provokes groans and guilt in non-exercisers. Once you find a type of exercise that suits you and your lifestyle, the benefits invariably outweigh the extra effort – and it is never too late to start.

Bodies are designed to be used, but many women lead sedentary lives with labour-saving devices at home, transport to work and physically undemanding desk jobs. Some people believe that it is natural to exercise less as they get older but this is a big mistake. It has been suggested that the need for exercise actually *increases* with age. Many of the aches and pains which are associated with age can be alleviated by exercise. One benefit that exercise gives is especially relevant to women: reducing the risk of osteoporosis.

Strengthen Your Bones

Young people should get plenty of exercise while their skeleton is still maturing but adults need to continue to exercise to maintain and strengthen their muscles and bone mass. The greater the bone mass you build up before

BENEFITS OF REGULAR EXERCISE

Exercise can:

- maintain and strengthen bone mass, reducing the risks of osteoporosis
- combat muscular aches and pains and stiffness and discourage the development of arthritis
- help to reduce blood pressure and protect against heart and arterial disease as well as lung disease
- help decrease body fat and reshape your body
- help you to sleep better without using pills
- improve the quality of your life by giving you a sense of well-being
- improve your posture
- give you more energy and stamina.

Most women feel better, healthier and even look better when they are exercising regularly.

you reach the menopause, the more protection you have against osteoporosis.

Athletes, cross-country runners, ballet dancers and weight-lifters have a higher than average bone mass. Professional tennis players develop stronger bones in their playing arm than casual tennis players of the same age. The type of exercise that is osteogenic – that helps prevent osteoporosis – should be vigorous and weight-bearing, involving pull and stress on the long bones of your body. Examples are aerobics, skipping and brisk walking. These exercises all include striking the feet on a hard surface. (It is important to remember to wear protective shoes, such as trainers, with this type of exercise.)

In a study comparing the effects of three types of regular exercise (practised three times a week) on bone mass, walking on a treadmill was more beneficial than bicycling or muscular exercise.[1] However, aerobic exercises and brisk walking have similar positive effects, and they might be more easily incorporated in your weekly routine. It is important to enjoy your exercise, so if you have more adventurous tastes, such as hang-gliding, water-skiing or tap-dancing, do pursue them.

Aerobic exercise is the type that puts demands on your heart and lungs – it makes you breathe more quickly and your heart beat faster. Whether the exercise you do is aerobic or not depends on your fitness and whether your pulse rate increases, and your ideal pulse rate depends on your age. Aerobic exercise which stimulates 65–80 per cent of your maximum heart rate is considered to be good for your bones. This means that if, after exercising for five to ten minutes, your pulse rate is within the range stated in the box below, you will have achieved aerobic exercise.[1]

PULSE RATE FOR AEROBIC EXERCISE

Age	65–80% of maximum pulse rate
Under 25	120 – 160
25 – 30	117 – 156
30 – 35	114 – 152
35 – 40	111 – 148
40 – 45	108 – 144
45 – 50	105 – 140
50 – 55	102 – 136
55 – 60	99 – 132
60 – 65	96 – 128
over 65	93 – 124

Aerobic exercise should be sustained for about five to ten minutes, depending on your level of fitness. If you do too much and become intolerably breathless it can be bad for you, especially if you are unfit. So gradually does it. Repeating the amount of aerobic exercise that is right for you two or three times a week will be good for your heart, lungs and circulation, and should help to protect you against osteoporosis. In a recent study of women aged between 32 and 78, thirty seconds of daily exercise (hand grips), produced significant increases in bone density (measured on their arms) after six weeks.[2]

A word of caution: before you embark on an exercise programme, particularly if you have been sedentary or bedridden for an extended period of time, seek advice from your doctor. He or she can suggest the type of activity that will be best for you. For example, if you have a history of heart disease or if you already have osteoporosis, jogging would not be suitable. It is also possible to exercise too much. Women who are highly athletic, such as marathon runners, can become amenorrhoeic (when their periods stop), which in itself leads to lowered oestrogen levels and bone loss. However, you have to do an awful lot of exercise for this to happen.

Walking, especially brisk walking, is a good form of aerobic exercise. It can be varied with strolling and you might prefer it if you dislike more formal exercise sessions. It can be really enjoyable – a time to think and to relax mentally. Keep a good straight posture and try to breathe from the depths of your lungs rather than with lots of short breaths. Start, perhaps, by walking to the shops rather than going in the car, or take a dog for regular walks. This, together with a general awareness of exercise, such as running upstairs and bending and stretching during daily activities, can be enough, and once established in your routine it will feel perfectly natural. Shirley, 49, preferred this type of exercise:

> I have my daily routines. I walk briskly to the shop every morning, then when I do my housework and gardening, which I love, I deliberately bend and stretch more than I need to. I work in the afternoons so I walk briskly all the way there and get the bus back. I always avoid lifts and run upstairs – it's surprising how much exercise this provides.

Exercise needs to be regular, this is why it is important to find something that fits with your lifestyle, so you can do it on a daily basis or about three times a week. It should also be enjoyable. Think about whether you prefer indoor or outdoor activities. Some women enjoy exercising alone, with the flexibility of using a video or cassette tape, while others like to attend a class or exercise with friends, which can be more fun. Is there a particular time of the day that you feel more energetic? Try several types of exercise before deciding on your fitness routine. Some women prefer a combined approach. Isabel, 42, described her routine:

> I go swimming once a week with two friends. I walk briskly to the shops about two to three times a week and I use an aerobics tape about twice a week. For me varying the exercise helps to fit it more naturally into my week. I recommend it!

Incidentally swimming is very good for muscles and for the cardiovascular system. Although it is not the type of exercise that prevents osteoporosis, it is very invigorating and relaxing.

From the point of view of osteoporosis the sooner you start exercising the better. Exercise is good for everyone but if you are at risk of osteoporosis, exercise can help you to prevent this problem. (To find out if you are at risk see page 57.) The results of recent studies suggest that women who exercise regularly *after* the menopause are less likely to suffer from osteoporosis.[2,3] If you are fit you will also probably be stronger and less vulnerable to falls and fractures.

Exercise and Well-Being

Exercise is known to promote a feeling of well-being and reduce symptoms of depression and anxiety. In my study, the women who took regular exercise before the menopause were less likely to be anxious, depressed or to have minor physical symptoms when they reached the menopause. So if the attraction of hormone replacement therapy is a 'mental tonic effect', you could try exercise instead. Maisie, 51, describes what exercise did for her:

I always used to be an active person but when I became depressed five years ago [this was due to a combination of family disputes and loss of a close friend] I just gradually gave up everything. It all seemed too much effort. As time passed and I began, with help, to sort out my problems, I was advised to take up some sort of exercise. I chose a dance exercise class but at first it was such an effort to get myself there. I went through the motions and came home. But after several weeks I started to enjoy it – I felt more able to do the exercises, and afterwards I became generally stronger and more confident. I still go to classes regularly and now it's more like a social event than hard work.

Exercise can also help you to sleep. If you have difficulty getting off because you feel tense and anxious and then feel tired during the day as a result, try exercises at home or a brisk walk in the late afternoon or early evening. It really does work. Sex is a form of exercise that can be relaxing or exhilarating – it can also serve as a remedy for insomnia.

It is not exactly known why exercise makes us feel good but there is fairly strong evidence to suggest that, after certain sorts of exercise, chemicals called endorphins are released which naturally produce a feeling of euphoria. Research studies show that it is short but sustained vigorous exercise, such as aerobics, that is associated with improvements in mood. Although many people feel more energetic straight after exercise, the major effects generally emerge after about ten weeks of regular exercise. So don't give up – you have a lot to gain and nothing to lose.

A Healthy Diet

What is healthy these days? The foods that I thought were good for me and my family apparently aren't. Avoiding pesticides and preservatives seems like a full-time job! *Susie, 47*

I think that women do suffer from a bad diet. This, coupled with extra stresses, I'm sure makes them have more problems such as PMT and depression. *Trish, 39*

Many health problems are caused or made worse by what we eat – heart disease, high blood pressure, bowel disorders and diabetes are a few examples. Many women say that they feel more energetic and calmer after improving their diet, as well as noticing improvements in their skin and hair. There is some evidence that menstrual problems and hot flushes can be relieved by certain changes in diet (see pages 128–30).[4]

Eating healthily usually means following a wholefood diet made up of food that is unrefined, unprocessed and is eaten raw or lightly cooked. Try to regularly eat a balanced combination of the following foods:

- Fresh fruits are rich in vitamins, minerals and fibre.
- Fresh vegetables, especially those that are dark green, are a good source of vitamins. Eat raw when you can, otherwise steam, using small amounts of water.
- Wholemeal breads and cereals and pulses, such as oats, rice, noodles, pasta, beans, nuts and seeds, provide dietary fibre and protein, as well as essential vitamins and minerals.
- Milk, cheese and yoghurt are vital because women need adequate supplies of calcium throughout life.
- Meat, fish and poultry and eggs are rich in protein. Vary your choice and include liver and oily fish as well as white fish.
- Drink water rather than soft drinks.

Try to cut down on the following and change some habits:

- Reduce your salt intake, as too much can increase blood pressure.

- Refined sugar in cakes, biscuits, cereals and sauces increases weight.
- Animal fats contain cholesterol which increases your chances of developing diseases of the heart and arteries. Try cooking without fat more often, or use vegetable-based oils such as corn or olive oil.
- Alcohol can be harmful if consumed excessively. Seek counselling and advice from your doctor if this is a problem for you (see page 165).
- Cut down on coffee.
- Stop smoking, or at the very least cut down.

Many women find that once they take the first step of thinking in terms of a healthy diet, their tastes also change, and they are less likely to want the cakes or chocolates that they had craved beforehand. This type of approach is very different to most slimming diets (although women will almost certainly lose weight with it if they were previously overweight) because it is caring rather than punishing. This was the case for Beth, 46, who has always viewed her weight as a problem:

I had tried most types of slimming diets but I usually gave up, because I just felt hungry all the time. I recently changed my doctor to one who is particularly interested in eating problems. She recommended a fibre-rich natural diet. It suits me so much bétter because I can actually eat a full plate of food without feeling guilty.

Women are often prone to suffer from self-hate when it comes to food – many eat for comfort and then despise themselves afterwards for it. If you have a particular eating problem, such as anorexia nervosa or bulimia (bingeing then vomiting after eating), do seek help. There are now better services available for women who suffer from these problems. (For counselling contacts see page 167.)

For most women the message is to eat sensibly and get to know how much food your body needs. The amount needed will probably reduce with age, but this will also depend upon how much exercise you take.

More and more restaurants and canteens now offer wholefood menus, and many people manage to stick to this regime at home. If you are restricted by time, salads are quick and easy to prepare and so is pasta.

Some health experts recommend taking supplements, often in high doses. Others claim that we can obtain all the vitamins and minerals we need from a good diet. This is still a matter for debate but it makes sense, if for example your lifestyle sometimes prevents you from eating regular amounts of good foods, to take a daily multivitamin and mineral tablet.

Calcium and Your Bones

There is one mineral that you do need to make sure you are getting enough: calcium. It is estimated that premenopausal women need about 1,000 mgs of calcium per day for healthy bones, while for postmenopausal women the requirement increases to around 1,400 mgs. The average British woman only consumes an estimated 500 to 800 mgs of calcium, and in the US the intake varies between 450 and 600 mgs for women aged 40 to 65 years. Therefore many women need to increase their intake by 100 per cent.

There is some disagreement among experts about the role of calcium in the prevention of osteoporosis and the value of calcium supplements (tablets). It is important to build up strong bones before the menopause to protect against osteoporosis and this process requires an *adequate* calcium intake throughout life, but most experts believe that the majority of women can obtain enough calcium with only slight dietary changes. It is more important to stay within the recommended levels *throughout* life, particularly during the years that bones are growing. The British Nutrition Foundation suggests that, 'an adequate supply of calcium in the diet up to the age of 30 is more important in preventing it (osteoporosis) than calcium tablets later in life'.

So, educate your daughters, and give them lots of milk and cheese.

Generally, for various reasons, women often do not eat calcium-rich foods. In a North American study of women engaged in an exercise programme to prevent osteoporosis, only 12 per cent were taking in the recommended amounts of calcium.[5] Their concern about weight gain and constipation, dislike of certain dairy products and lactose intolerance (allergy to dairy products) discouraged them from eating enough calcium-rich foods. Yoghurt is often tolerated when milk products are not, and now many women are choosing to drink skimmed milk which has all the benefits of calcium, with fewer calories.

If you are a vegetarian and you avoid meat, poultry and fish but allow dairy products, then your diet is likely to provide you with enough calcium. There is even some evidence that a high intake of protein might contribute to bone loss. So a vegetarian diet like this may put you at an advantage with regard to healthy bones, provided that you have adequate amounts of dairy products. However, a vegan or strict vegetarian diet, in which all dairy foods are avoided, can be low in calcium and vitamin D. An easy solution is to use soya milk that has been fortified with calcium and vitamins.

The combination of diet and exercise is vital. Recent evidence suggests that for exercise to help prevent osteoporosis you must have enough calcium in your diet.

How Can I Get Enough Calcium?

Skimmed milk and yoghurts are probably the best source of calcium, but sardines, sprats, pilchards, nuts, dried fruit, leafy green vegetables, cheese and eggs are also calcium-rich. If you need them, calcium supplements are fairly cheap to buy, and skimmed milk is supplemented with calcium.

Dr Morris Notelovitz, Director of the Center of Cli-

GOOD SOURCES OF CALCIUM[6]

Food	Amount	Calcium (mgs)
Cow's milk	¼ pint	180
Skimmed milk	¼ pint	195
Natural yoghurt	3 ½ ozs	180
Cheddar cheese	2 ozs	400
Camembert cheese	2 ozs	190
Parmesan cheese	1 oz	305
Tinned salmon	3 ½ ozs	195
Tinned sardines	3 ½ ozs	460
Raw oysters	3 ½ ozs	190
Dried figs	3 ½ ozs	280
Muesli	3 ½ ozs	200
Tofu (bean curd)	3 ½ ozs	507
Spinach (boiled)	3 ½ ozs	600
Watercress (raw)	2 ozs	110

macteric Studies in Florida, and advocate of non-hormonal management of the menopause, stresses that the calcium requirement is needed consistently on a daily basis. He says, 'As with exercise, individuals need to be given the option of meeting this need by whatever means are convenient, acceptable and affordable.'

Joyce, 42, has a family history of osteoporosis and she is careful to have enough calcium in her diet. She has found a compromise between dietary and supplementary calcium:

When I am organised and take lunch with me to work and when I am at home at weekends, I do manage with diet alone. But if I am away on business or end up working late and not eating properly, I take a calcium tablet. It's reassuring to have them, I usually carry them around with me.

There are several forms of calcium supplements – calcium carbonate is usually recommended since it contains more calcium (40%) than calcium lactate (13%) and calcium glutamate (9%). Calcium is not much good without vitamin D which is required to help the body to absorb calcium properly and some calcium supplements include vitamin D. But too much vitamin D can be harmful and lead to an increase in the amount of calcium excreted. So at the moment it seems that the average intake of vitamin D should not exceed 1,000 international units per day (a rate of measure) and most people get this from sunlight. Only very elderly people probably need a supplement. If in doubt, seek advice from your doctor. Bone meal and dolomite supplements (containing calcium) are also available, but these do contain small amounts of lead, a substance which most people would wisely wish to avoid.

Probably the best approach is to keep a rough note of your intake of calcium for a couple of weeks. Then, if necessary, try to increase it by regulating your diet. This should not be too difficult for most women. But if you are lactose intolerant, or you dislike many of the foods that contain calcium, try supplements. It would be wise to monitor your calcium intake again while including the supplements. Excessive levels of calcium can cause kidney stones, so women who already suffer from kidney stones or hyperparathyroidism should not take supplements. The experts cannot agree on whether other mineral supplements, such as magnesium and phosphorus, are necessary. On balance the evidence suggests that they are not.

MAKING THE EFFORT

Preparation for the menopause – a natural approach to alleviate menopausal and postmenopausal problems – has immediate and long-term benefits for your health and well-being, and it is safe and free from side-effects. But will we make the effort? We live in a materialistic and medicating society in which fast, easy solutions to problems are sought and bought.

The major disadvantage of a natural approach to the menopause is it has to depend on two unreliable human qualities: will-power and persistence. This is why the changes in your lifestyle must be carefully planned to adapt to your needs as much as possible. The message is: do what you can. For example, if the best levels of exercise suggested here are too much for you, start with a once weekly exercise and see how you feel. A healthy diet need not take a lot of preparation and you don't need to resort to instant packet foods if you are busy; fruit and wholemeal sandwiches are quick, and far healthier.

Experience has shown that people can and will change aspects of their lives if they are properly informed, so the task of changing attitudes and challenging myths has an important part to play. Whether we are going to stick to exercise or non-smoking programmes depends on a delicate balance between effort and pay-off, as well as understanding the benefits. I believe that we can do it. Many people have already changed to healthier diets and have stopped smoking, and consumers are demanding organically-grown foods as a result of their distrust of modern agricultural methods and the food industry. Exercise is now much more fashionable than it was twenty years ago.

In an attempt to find out whether an osteoporosis prevention education programme would influence women to alter their lifestyle, researchers at the Center for Climacteric Studies in Florida sent an educational package to over 700 randomly selected women.[7] These women were also offered bone densiometry scanning (which assesses bone mass). When they were contacted a year later, over 80 per cent of the women who had been showing signs of bone loss had significantly altered their lifestyle.

SELF-HELP OR MEDICAL SERVICES?

By seeking information and making the effort you can prepare yourself for the menopause. Of course this would be so much easier if the right facilities were already in place. We need to develop centres, groups and networks where women can get information, share experiences and give and receive support on all aspects of the menopause. You are far more likely to succeed in altering your lifestyle or diet if you are part of a group, rather than being dependent only on self-motivation. At the same time groups are not everyone's cup of tea – you may prefer to start exercising, or discussing the menopause, with one or two close friends.

Several menopause self-help groups do exist in Britain (see page 163), offering a range of facilities including groups, workshops, information and counselling; and if you are keen to set up a group in your area, contact one of these groups for advice. They can also be of use to women in their thirties and forties by encouraging them to challenge attitudes and take preventative action before they reach the menopause.

We need to campaign for better health care for pre- and postmenopausal women too. Contact your local Community Health Council to find out about the services in your area. With cuts in the NHS since the late 1970s, established menopause clinics are having difficulty getting funds (see page 169 for list of clinics). But a menopause facility in a Well Woman clinic, for example, offering preventative information, advice and support for women – whether they are menopausal, prematurely menopausal or postmenopausal – could be of enormous benefit, as well as being cost-effective to the health service in the long-term.

7

Help Yourself

Many women dislike being dependent on medication and, whether you are one of them or not, it makes sense to try to reduce the symptoms related to the menopause yourself, before considering treatments such as hormone replacement therapy (HRT). Some women decide that they do not need treatment. Even if your symptoms are very troublesome, there are simple and practical ways to alleviate hot flushes and night sweats, and vaginal dryness is commonly helped by non-hormonal methods. The main measures – exercise and diet – recommended to help prevent osteoporosis have already been described in Chapter 6.

Obviously it is best to stick to a good diet and regular exercise throughout the menopausal years and beyond. Remember that physical activity can help to strengthen your muscles and your bones, and it will help you to feel better both physically and emotionally. Homoeopathic or herbal remedies have helped some women through the menopause, while others find vitamins useful. For women who have severe symptoms and for whom HRT is not advisable, alternative methods are the answer.

SELF-HELP

For Hot Flushes and Night Sweats

- Use cotton clothes and sheets rather than artificial fibres.
- Wear layers of light clothing so that you can easily remove one or two.
- Open windows in stuffy rooms; sit next to a window at work. If you can, invest in a small desk fan.
- Try to cut down or, better still, stop smoking, as this increases sweating.
- Cut down on sugar for the same reason.
- Reduce stimulants such as tea, coffee, hot spicy foods and alcohol. All these can trigger flushes.
- During a flush, cool down by going to an open window or putting your wrists under cold running water. A cold shower may be helpful, especially in hot weather.
- At night use thin, layered bedcovers. Keep the window open. A drink of water can help. If you are woken up by sweats, try not to worry about missing sleep – read for a while, try to relax, and your body will probably adjust to give you the sleep you need. Remember that we need less sleep as we get older anyway.
- Don't panic, and don't fight a hot flush. Keep calm and try to relax. Don't be ashamed of hot flushes – they are normal and millions of other women are sharing your experience. If you want to stop what you are doing to cool down, do so. Try telling people what you are doing and why you are doing it. Be brave and educate others.

- Relaxation is one of the best ways to reduce hot flushes. Learn a simple method of muscular relaxation, using a tape (available at health shops) or by following the instructions here. Breathe slowly from your stomach. Practise until you can relax quickly and easily when you are sitting down. Learning to relax is like learning any new skill – you need to practise. In two North American studies women who suffered from hot flushes were taught relaxation in six to ten half-hour sessions. The frequency of their flushes reduced by 80 per cent and some women learnt to stop hot flushes by relaxing when they felt one coming on. This treatment is good for your health, it is easy to learn and it is safe and free from side-effects. Spread the word! It is an ideal therapy for women to learn together in small groups.

- Biofeedback and autogenic training are specific methods that can be used to control bodily temperature before or during a flush. Biofeedback enables people to become aware of physical changes in the body, such as muscle tension or temperature, by amplifying electronic signals and feeding them back, usually in the form of a sound. But equipment for biofeedback is expensive and relaxation is probably as effective. Autogenic training is a method of increasing control over bodily systems by self-suggestion. When you relax you can try suggesting to yourself that your hands are warm and that your head and chest feel calm and cool.

- These techniques should be combined with a general campaign to reduce stress and, if you can, avoid certain situations that you find bring on your hot flushes. By monitoring your flushes and activities you can

RELAXATION INSTRUCTIONS

By systematically tensing and relaxing your muscles they will relax more fully. You can concentrate on your breathing to calm your thoughts. Sit in a comfortable armchair, wearing loose clothing and no shoes. Free yourself from interruptions for about twenty minutes.

- First focus on the feelings in your body. Notice if you are particularly tense anywhere.
- Tense your arms and hands by making tight fists and bending your arms for a few seconds. Hold them tight – then relax. Let them drop down on the arms of the chair. Notice the feelings in your arms and hands as the muscles relax and imagine the relaxation spreading down from your shoulders to your fingertips, as if it would be an effort to move them.
- Next tense your shoulders taking a deep breath and lifting your shoulders up and back. Tense and relax as before. This time also concentrate on your breathing. It should be passive, gentle, even breathing (as it usually feels just before you go to sleep), from your stomach rather than your chest. Just notice your breathing and let yourself relax further each time you breathe out.
- Repeat, tensing your stomach by making the muscles tight. Relax muscles and concentrate on breathing.
- Repeat for legs and feet. Stretch out your legs, tensing all muscles. Relax and concentrate on breathing.
- Give yourself 5–10 minutes at the end to let your whole body relax. Feel yourself sinking into the chair. At this stage some women choose a relaxing image to think about, such as watching a river, sitting in a garden, floating in a pool, or you can just notice your breathing. Practise at least once a day and you will learn to relax more quickly.

learn what precipitates flushes for you – woman differ a lot in this respect. For example, for one woman it was being the passenger in a car rather than driving herself. Several have said that flushes increase when they are time pressured or have too much to do.

Reduce stress by delegating and saying no to things you do not want to do, and by not overloading yourself with commitments. Put yourself, your health and well-being first. If cooking over a hot oven or lifting heavy objects make flushes worse, ask someone else to help or cut out these activities if you can.

For Vaginal Dryness

- If you are in a sexual relationship, talk about vaginal dryness with your partner. Take longer over foreplay so that you are fully aroused before penetration. If you do not want penetration, because it might hurt, say so. Instead, try love-making without penetration.
- Use a vaginal lubricant such as KY jelly, which is widely available from chemists.
- Masturbation can also help, whether you are in a sexual relationship or not. Regular vaginal lubrication before and during the menopause does seem to maintain vaginal moisture.
- Pelvic floor exercises, which are taught as part of antenatal care, tone up the pelvic floor muscles and increase the blood flow to the genitals, thereby keeping the vagina moist and healthy. They also help prevent and ease stress incontinence. Exercise these muscles by pulling up the muscles which form a figure of eight around the vagina and anus. Try to pass water and stop yourself. Then release the muscles, and repeat

several times. One woman found it helpful to imagine the muscles were like a lift, going up quickly and coming down in gradual stages. You can practise these exercises anywhere. No one will know.

- Some women have found that natural, live yoghurt applied inside the vagina is soothing and can ward off vaginal infections and decrease dryness.

General Self-help

After caring for others, often for many years, and working either in or out of the home or both, the menopause is the stage of life during which women deserve to focus the caring on *themselves*. Ask yourself the following questions:

- Do I try to live up to an unrealistic ideal? Am I trying to be superhuman?
- Do I usually blame myself when things go wrong?
- Do I tend to be the victim in relationships?
- Do I often tell myself 'I should . . .'?
- Is there a strict parent in my head being critical of me?

If you answer yes to any of these questions, then be more aware of these tendencies. Notice the ways that you think about yourself and question them. Ask yourself, 'Why should I? Who is telling me to do that?' or 'Why do I feel guilty, as if it is my responsibility?' Try to free yourself a little from restrictions. Women frequently tell me that they don't go out or do things for themselves because they think that their partner or family will disapprove. However, when they do take charge of their lives and begin to do these things, they are often proved wrong.

While some women are trapped in unhealthy relationships, others admit that they are their own worst enemy.

Let your body tell you what it needs. Improve your diet and make time to relax and exercise. Feeding yourself well is a good way of starting to care for yourself. Do you bother to eat well when you are on your own?

When she set aside an hour a day purely for herself, Margie, 47, alternated relaxation and aerobic exercises, followed by a soothing hot bath. She described it as 'heaven' and wondered why she had not let herself have this time before:

> I had to be really strict with myself at first and was tempted to do all sorts of other things instead. Now I've trained myself to switch off for that hour. I take the phone off the hook and don't answer the door!

Exercise and relaxation can also be a social activity if you prefer. Yoga and exercise classes are widely available in the evening and often in the daytime. Find the method or type of exercise that suits your lifestyle, whether at a regular time with others or using a tape at home.

One of the problems that some women feel during the menopause is that their bodies have changed and are not as dependable as before.

> My body feels out of control. It is unpredictable and I feel as though it is generally vulnerable. *Iris*, 49

Exercise and relaxation helped Iris to regain a sense of control over her body. She began to look after herself instead of just feeling annoyed about the physical changes, like hot flushes, that were taking place.

Give yourself time to think about stresses, talk to other people and try to solve problems. Assess your priorities – your health and happiness should be high on the list.

Self-help Groups

Talking to other women can be enjoyable and stimulating. Menopause self-help groups provide an excellent opportunity to gain information and encouragement, as well as a different perspective on your own problems and a place to start talking openly about the menopause. There is as yet no national network in Britain, but there are several well-established groups (see page 164). You can find out by asking at your local Community Health Council, Well Woman Clinic, Health Education Office or the Women's Health Information Centre (WHIC). For addresses of the WHIC and other women's organisations that might be helpful if you are looking for contacts or wanting to start a group yourself, see page 163.

There is no reason why you cannot start your own group with about five to ten women. You could advertise or just spread the word. Costs are minimal if, for example, you take turns in hosting a two-hour meeting each week or fortnight. Each meeting could focus on a previously agreed topic or you could take turns to lead the discussions.

Vitamins, Minerals and Supplements

Vitamin B6
Women taking certain oestrogens and progestogens may be deficient in vitamin B6 and this can cause depression

and tiredness. So women taking HRT could try B6 if they suffer from these symptoms. If you have premenstrual symptoms before the menopause you might also benefit from B6. It is found in whole grains, milk, yeast, egg yolk, rice and bran.

Vitamin E

Many women have found that vitamin E helps relieve hot flushes and night sweats. Start by taking 100 international units daily for a month. If this does not work, increase the dose to between 300 and 600 international units per day for two to three months. If the symptoms subside, gradually reduce your intake over several months, until you are taking the lowest dose and it is still having a positive effect. It takes several weeks to take effect, so be patient. Once you have found the best dose for you, stop taking it for a month every now and again. Women also claim improvements in vaginal lubrication when taking vitamin E.

It is best taken with vitamin C and selenium, which help it to be absorbed. It is found naturally in wheatgerm oil, and in wheat germ and whole-grains (especially oatmeal), in corn, soyabeans and peanuts. Vitamin E does contain small amounts of oestrogen, so if oestrogens are not advisable for you, because of breast cancer, for example, your doctor will probably not recommend it.

Avoid vitamin E if you have heart problems, high blood pressure or diabetes or ask your doctor.

Calcium

During and after the menopause the recommended daily intake of calcium is 1400 mgs. It can be taken in pill form but it is also found in milk, yoghurt, cheese, sardines and watercress. (See page 115 for further details.)

Efamol (oil of evening primrose)

This is now a popular alternative for premenstrual symptoms and many women swear by it. It is also thought to help when you are under stress, as well as during the hormonal upheavals before and during the menopause. Doses of one or two 500 mg capsules taken two or three times daily are usually recommended, but Efamol is expensive so you could try a smaller dose first. It is safe to take in large doses.

Ginseng

While commonly taken as a tonic or general panacea, ginseng has been used with vitamin E to alleviate hot flushes, night sweats, headaches and palpitations in menopausal women. Siberian ginseng, rather than Korean ginseng, is the one recommended for hot flushes and between 400 and 600 mgs of the dried root should be taken every day, or it can be taken in capsule form. Buy it from a reputable dealer and seek advice from a herbalist about the best dose for you. Also, you might seek your doctor's advice if you are not supposed to use oestrogens for health reasons, as ginseng might contain oestrogen in small amounts.

Which supplements, if any, you choose to take and whether you take them in tablet form or whether you modify your diet to get them that way, will depend on many factors, including your lifestyle. If you are busy and prefer not to spend time working out your daily rations of various foods, then pills might be your choice. For example, you could begin with a multivitamin, which will include the essential vitamins and minerals you need, plus calcium. However, if hot flushes or premenstrual symptoms become a problem for you then you could move on to one of the more specific supplements such as B6, Efamol or vitamin E.

Vitamin and mineral tablets especially for menopausal women are now available from chemists and health food shops and they contain combinations of supplements in one tablet or capsule, usually vitamins and calcium. Be wary of products with unrealistic claims. An adequate supply of calcium after the menopause is advisable, but this will not *cure* osteoporosis.

Research on dietary remedies continues. An element called 'boron' is being hailed as 'the natural HRT' in the USA because studies suggest that it not only helps women retain more calcium and magnesium, but it also increases oestrogen levels. Food sources of boron include apples, pears, tomatoes, prunes, raisins, dates, honey and cow's milk. It is also available as a supplement. However, until further research is carried out we cannot know for sure whether these claims are justified. Women are using all these supplements on a trial basis and many do seem to find something to suit their own particular needs.

Many of the vitamins and minerals mentioned in this chapter can be prescribed on the NHS. Talk to your GP if your symptoms are causing you distress and you wish to try particular supplements or vitamins.

ALTERNATIVE THERAPIES

If you make the changes in diet and exercise which have been suggested so far, you may well feel generally healthier and have fewer symptoms during the menopause. For specific symptoms that persist, such as headaches, hot flushes, tiredness and tension, you might want to try alternative therapies. It is crucial, however, that you see your doctor first to get a proper diagnosis, so that you can rule out serious disease. For example, if you have a breast lump or experience vaginal bleeding after the menopause or following intercourse, you should seek medical advice.

Homoeopathy

Homoeopathic medicine is based on treating the illness or symptoms by prescribing a carefully matched substance. A remedy is chosen on the basis of the similar symptoms it would produce if the homoeopathic medicine were given to a healthy person. This approach will involve an assessment of your physical and emotional well-being, as well as your lifestyle, and your homoeopath will need to know, in detail, about the exact quality of your symptoms.

Treatment is made up of small doses of natural substances from herbal, animal, mineral and metallic sources. Improvement can be rapid, sometimes within twenty-four hours. For menopausal symptoms, nux vomica, sepia and lachesis might be chosen. While it is possible to diagnose and treat yourself, this is not advisable as there are subtle distinctions between the different symptoms and their appropriate remedies. If you are interested in this approach, contact a registered homoeopath (see page 167).

Herbal Remedies

These are derived from natural substances such as plants, seeds, roots or barks – some are centuries old and predate modern medicine. Herbal remedies can be very potent; they are administered in various forms such as infusions, powders, ointments or linaments. Like homoeopathy, the whole person is considered in the diagnosis and treatment and it is probably best to see a qualified herbal practitioner (see page 168), rather than to try to treat yourself. Sometimes a change in your diet is all that is suggested, but if you are prescribed herbal remedies, then regular follow-up visits are necessary to check on your progress. It can take some time, from weeks to months, to ease severe symptoms using this approach.

Acupuncture

By stimulating certain acupuncture points on the body (called energy channels or meridians), with specially designed needles, this therapy aims to rebalance bodily forces (Yin and Yang) and hence alleviate symptoms. Acupuncture is commonly used for pain relief, but it is also claimed that hot flushes, night sweats, menstrual irregularities and vaginal soreness and irritation, as well as general tiredness, can respond to this treatment. Again it is important to see a qualified practitioner, preferably someone who is registered with one of the recognised acupuncture organisations (see page 168).

Naturopathy

This approach helps the body to heal itself, using its natural mechanisms and without recourse to medicaments. Various treatments such as diets, exercises and massage are used, as well as herbs. If you are interested in this approach, see page 168 for a list of registered naturopaths.

You can see from this chapter that a wide range of treatment and preventative approaches are available to women who wish to alleviate their symptoms during the menopause. These methods have not received the same amount of publicity, in newspapers and magazines, as the medical treatment for menopausal women, which is hormone replacement therapy.

8

Hormone Replacement Therapy

Women are divided on the subject of hormone replacement therapy (HRT). Over the past ten years there has been a great deal of research into HRT, its side-effects, risks and benefits. But it is increasingly difficult to gain a clear picture of the pros and cons of HRT because the findings of one study will usually conflict with another. When I asked women in their thirties and forties what they felt about HRT their opinions varied:

It's a good thing for women.

I'm against drugs, if at all possible. After all we've read about the contraceptive pill, I'd be reluctant to put myself at risk again.

It sounds to me like another example of women's problems being medicalised – surely it should be a natural process.

Doctors also have differing opinions; while some GPs

are reluctant to prescribe HRT, others, such as Frances, 38, are keener:

> I offer it to menopausal women if they have physical or emotional symptoms during the menopause. I intend to take it myself for its general effects on skin and health.

WHAT IS HRT?

The hormones used in hormone replacement therapy are either synthetic oestrogens, or a mixture of natural and horse oestrogens, or natural oestrogens. The most commonly prescribed oestrogen is a mixed or 'conjugated' oestrogen derived from the urine of pregnant mares (hence its brand name Premarin). Synthetic oestrogens are more potent than conjugated oestrogens, and conjugated oestrogens are more potent than natural oestrogens. Human oestrogens are not used in 'natural' oestrogens largely because supplies of human oestrogens cannot meet the demand for HRT. Instead, they are made in the laboratory, but they are very similar to naturally occurring oestrogens. Synthetic oestrogens, which were used in the contraceptive pill, are different in chemical structure and are not like human oestrogens.

Because oestrogens increase the likelihood of women developing cancer of the womb, most doctors now prescribe a *progestogen* for the last twelve or thirteen days of the month as well to reduce this risk. When women who have not had a hysterectomy take oestrogen and progestogen they menstruate even though they are postmenopausal. Although the ratio of oestrogens and progestogens given roughly mirrors the general balance of hormones before the menopause, it is unlikely to reproduce the finely-tuned balance of your premenopausal hormones.

It is estimated that between 5 and 8 per cent of menopausal and postmenopausal women in Britain are taking HRT, compared with about 20 to 30 per cent in the USA. In both countries the figures are rising.

There are different doses and different ways of taking HRT: orally in pills, with skin patches, implants or creams (see page 150). The most common regime in Britain and the USA has been conjugated oestrogens taken orally (Premarin), but skin patches containing natural oestrogens are increasingly popular with doctors and they are preferred by many women. Scandinavian women tend to choose natural oestrogens while French women apparently prefer oestrogen creams.

You will find that doctors tend to prefer one method over another but, providing there are no medical reasons against a particular method, the choice should be yours. As we shall see later, the risks and side-effects of oestrogens are, to some extent, dependent upon the oestrogen type, dosage and the way it is taken. Patches, pills and creams offer women more control over the dose and the ability to stop treatment themselves if they wish. Further details of types of HRT available, the doses and what each contains are given on page 161.

BENEFITS OF HRT

Hot Flushes and Night Sweats

Hot flushes and night sweats are alleviated or stop altogether after HRT. These symptoms will eventually stop on their own but for a few women they can be distressing and interfere with normal life. HRT probably works by stabilising oestrogen levels, rather than by replacing oestrogen. Treatment is usually recommended for about two years. It is important to stop HRT gradually, over a period of nine months, because symptoms can recur as the oestrogen in the body is reduced.

Vaginal Dryness

Vaginal dryness is associated with lower oestrogen levels and it can be helped by HRT. But if the symptom is caused by an unsatisfactory sexual relationship then of course HRT will not be a magical cure. Vaginal creams such as oestriol can be applied locally, in small doses, to reduce the possibility of health risks. Because vaginal dryness can be a persistent problem, some women continue to use HRT as a treatment for many years. However, ordinary lubricants can be effective if long-term treatment does not appeal to you (see page 124).

Osteoporosis

Osteoporosis is the thinning of the bones which can lead to fractures in later life and it can be prevented, to some extent, by HRT. But HRT does not put strength back into the bones, nor does it cure osteoporosis. If you are at risk of osteoporosis (see page 57), experts estimate that, by taking HRT at the onset of the menopause, for five years, you can reduce the risk of bone fractures that might follow by half. Some doctors recommend continued treatment for this for ten to twenty years. However, it is thought that there are few benefits to the bones if HRT is started too late, for example after the age of 65.

Heart Disease and Strokes

The number of strokes and the rate of heart disease increase in postmenopausal women (see page 60). There is some evidence to suggest that HRT might prevent the development of heart diseases. But at the moment we cannot know for certain since adding progestogens to the HRT regime might negate oestrogen's positive effects.

Emotional Problems

We have already established the fact that emotional problems do not necessarily *increase* in menopausal women (see Chapter 4). Distress during the menopausal years is caused primarily by personal or social reasons, rather than lack of oestrogen. Yet HRT is, in some medical circles, being regarded as a panacea, not only for hot flushes but also for more general life problems. Two of Britain's leading gynaecologists and advocates of HRT have written in a textbook for medical students:

> Because oestrogen therapy can prevent many physical, psychological and even marital problems, with a particularly useful effect on depression, libido, the skeleton and the incidence of heart attacks, the practice of 'weaning off' after a few years does not make much sense.[1]

However, there is no conclusive evidence that HRT has a direct effect on mood, sex life or appearance, other than by relieving hot flushes or vaginal dryness. In fact, in the

USA, a warning is inserted into each packet of HRT, on the recommendation of the Federal Government's Food and Drug Administration, advising that it should *not* be used as a treatment for emotional problems.

DISADVANTAGES OF HRT

Health Risks

Endometrial Cancer

Endometrial cancer, or cancer of the lining of the womb, was one of the first worrying consequences of HRT. When oestrogens were initially prescribed in the 1960s and 1970s they were given alone or 'unopposed' by progestogens. Because oestrogen stimulates the growth of the lining of the womb, it can trigger the development of cancer and, during the 1970s, rates of this type of cancer increased, particularly in the US where oestrogens were widely prescribed.

Progestogens (synthetic progesterone), added for the last twelve or thirteen days each month, cause a breakdown of the lining of the womb and a monthly bleed for three to five days, and prevent the growth of cancer of the womb. Combined oestrogen and progestogen treatment is standard in Britain today for women who have not had a hysterectomy. (Women who have had a hysterectomy are usually prescribed oestrogen alone because they are not at risk of endometrial cancer, having had their wombs removed.) In the USA many doctors still prefer to prescribe oestrogen alone because progestogens, while preventing cancer of the womb, might counteract the possible benefits of oestrogen to the heart and circulation.

Breast Cancer

Breast cancer is the most common form of cancer in women and the likelihood of breast cancer rises throughout a woman's life. It is therefore very common in her postmenopausal years. The incidence of breast cancer is much higher in the western world. In western Europe, Australia and the US it is 86, 67 and 91 per 100,000 women respectively. This is compared with 6 and 8 per 100,000 women in China and East Africa.

Certain types of breast cancer are stimulated by oestrogen and therefore grow more quickly when oestrogens are circulating in the body, but the link between HRT and breast cancer is uncertain and a matter of controversy. While some studies show no change in development of it, others do show an increased risk. In the short term, hormone replacement therapy is thought to be relatively safe, but with long-term use over a period of six to ten years there is evidence from several studies to suggest a modest increase in risk. One of these studies found that the chances of developing breast cancer were raised by as much as 30 per cent after ten years of having the therapy.[2] However, as with most forms of cancer, other risk factors, such as family history, smoking, obesity and possibly the use of some types of contraceptive pills, will also be important.

The effects of progestogens on breast cancer are unknown. So far it is unclear whether they have a positive or a negative influence.

Thrombosis and Hypertension

Synthetic oestrogens, such as ethinyloestradiol, which form the basis of most contraceptive pills, are associated with thrombosis and hypertension, especially in women who are obese (as defined by their doctor, rather than just overweight), smoke or who have varicose veins. Women who are prescribed high doses of synthetic hormones are therefore at greater risk of thrombosis and hypertension. Conjugated equine oestrogens (Premarin) are safer, but they are not as safe as natural oestrogens. To complicate matters further, oestrogen can also have a positive effect on the cardiovascular system by dilating the blood vessel walls, and this might counteract its negative effects to some extent. Nevertheless women who are at risk of heart problems or strokes are advised not to take synthetic or equine oestrogens.

The way oestrogen is prescribed is also important in determining its risks. In the liver oestrogen works to activate certain proteins, some of which increase blood pressure and blood clotting. Oestrogens taken orally pass through the liver, but oestrogens implanted under the skin or applied in skin patches bypass the liver. Therefore certain risks, including thrombosis and hypertension, are reduced with the non-oral methods. At the same time, however, by avoiding the liver the possible positive effects of oestrogen on the cardiovascular system (causing heart attacks and strokes) are lessened.

Gallstones

Oestrogens increase a woman's chances of developing gall bladder disease; they can also aggravate existing gallstones – a common problem for women in their fifties and sixties. Since the effect of oestrogen on gall bladder function also takes place in the liver, women who have gallstones and want to take HRT should use very small doses, in the form of patches, creams or implants of oestrogen.

Fibroids and Endometriosis

Fibroids and endometriosis (overgrowth of the lining of the womb into the surrounding pelvic area) can be made worse by HRT because it stimulates the growth of the lining of the womb. This means that fibroids might increase in size, and endometriosis might spread. If you have either close monitoring is essential, and you should stop taking HRT if there is any indication that the problem is getting worse.

SIDE-EFFECTS OF HRT

Some women have no problems with HRT, while others suffer from various side-effects and stop the treatment as a result. A common, unwelcome effect is the return of monthly periods – most women over 50 don't relish periods, although some do not mind: of the women I talked to, those in their late fifties and sixties were more inclined to dislike the fact that they would go on needing sanitary protection. For some women the progestogens cause premenstrual-type symptoms such as tension, depression and bloating. Other side-effects include:

- fluid retention
- nausea and vomiting
- abdominal cramping
- breast tenderness
- weight gain
- irritability
- leg cramps.

Doctors will usually advise that most of these problems

are part of the body's initial adjustment to treatment, and expect them to disappear after two to three months. But obviously if they are unpleasant or severe, then the dose should be reduced, changed or the treatment stopped.

WHAT ARE WOMEN'S EXPERIENCES OF HRT?

Beatrice is 53. She has been taking HRT, in tablet form, for two years. She initially went to her doctor because of intense and frequent hot flushes and because she felt generally tired and stressed by problems at home:

> I feel much better on the treatment. The flushes have practically disappeared and, because I'm sleeping better, and am less tired, I have more patience with my daughter. I am a bit worried about what I will be like when I stop taking it – whether I am really better or not.

It is sometimes difficult to know whether hot flushes have really come to an end, or whether they will recur when you stop taking HRT. One answer is to gradually reduce the HRT to find out whether your hot flushes have stopped.

Paula, 47, has had continued HRT by implantation since her hysterectomy and oopherectomy (removal of the ovaries) six years ago:

> I can feel when the implant is running out because the hot flushes return. It seems to be happening more quickly and I need another one after three months rather than six months.

This can happen with implants, especially when high doses are used. In this case Paula's oestrogen levels were not particularly low and the implant had not run out, but her body had become sensitive to small reductions, resulting in the re-emergence of her symptoms. I have met a few women who need repeated high doses to maintain the benefits of HRT. They feel that HRT helps to give them energy and vitality. But they may be experiencing the 'mental tonic' effect – a physiological 'high' that sometimes occurs when oestrogens are taken in high doses. It is as if their bodies have become dependent upon these amounts of HRT. If this happens to you, try to reduce the oestrogen doses gradually, with the help of your doctor.

Terry, 53, swears by HRT, 'Since taking HRT I feel on top of the world, my skin feels better and people think I'm in my 40s.' And many women find that despite some side-effects, the benefits are worth it. Laura, now 48, had her menopause in her early forties:

My symptoms were so overwhelming I would have done anything to feel better: I had hot flushes, night sweats and I couldn't sleep well, and I was very low about the whole thing. I felt shattered for weeks before I started HRT. I have had to change the dose, but now I have patches, which seem to suit me. When I take the norethisterone [a progestogen] I don't sleep very well and feel more tired and edgy, but overall I'm happy with the treatment.

Marjorie went to a menopause clinic when her hot flushes started and her periods became irregular. She was concerned about the future of her bones because her mother had severe osteoporosis which led to a hip fracture and long spells in hospital:

> I've been taking HRT for nine months now. It feels rather strange taking pills for a problem you do not have. In fact in other respects my menopause was fine – I didn't have bad hot flushes or anything. I'll persist with it for now but I do wonder how long I'll be happy to carry on having periods.

This is a problem. Making an effort to prevent something that you are not sure will happen takes considerable motivation and perseverance.

Nell, 52, found her menopause very difficult to accept, 'Since taking hormone therapy I have really forgotten that I'm menopausal. I like it, I feel good and having regular periods makes me feel younger.'

To find out more about women's reactions to HRT I contacted 200 women who attended the menopause clinic at a London teaching hospital. Eighty per cent had been prescribed HRT. The average duration of the treatment was two years but it varied considerably: some women stopped after six months, others after one or two years. After four years just less than half of them were still continuing with the treatment. About two-thirds of those given HRT were considered by the gynaecologist to have benefitted from it somehow (ranging from some to much improvement). One in ten stopped treatment because of side-effects (such as nausea, painful breasts and dislike of menstruation) and not wanting to take hormones, and a similar proportion either did not improve or did not return to the clinic. It was the women who first went to the clinic with primarily emotional problems (problems which predated the menopause or were caused by personal or social factors) who benefited least from HRT.

IS HRT SAFE FOR ME?

If you have or have had any of the following conditions, you may be advised against taking HRT:

- Breast cancer, or benign breast disease
- A family history of breast cancer
- Cancer of the lining of the womb (some doctors also exclude women with a history of cancer of the ovary and cervix)
- Deep vein thrombosis or serious blood clot
- Heart conditions such as angina or heart attack
- Liver disease
- High blood pressure
- Diabetes
- Gall bladder disease
- Fibroids
- Jaundice (this may recur with oestrogens)
- Obesity
- If you are a heavy cigarette smoker

IS HRT FOR YOU?

Certain groups of women are often advised to consider HRT either as a treatment or as a preventative measure:

- Women who have a premature menopause (usually meaning before the age of 45) either naturally or because of surgery, chiefly to prevent osteoporosis. However, premature menopause is sometimes caused by drug treatment for breast cancer (such as Tamoxifen) which precludes oestrogen as a therapy. These women could try alternative therapies (see Chapter 7).

- Women who have a strong family history of osteoporosis, or who consider themselves at risk, because of a combination of other factors, including a poor diet, smoking, lack of exercise, small stature, fair skin, certain medical conditions or treatments (see page 57).
- Women who have severe hot flushes or night sweats, and feel unable to cope with them.
- Women with severe vaginal dryness or frequent vaginal infections can be helped by local application of creams.

The decision whether to take HRT is a very personal one. You need to make a list of the possible risks for you and the potential benefits and you need to be accurate about your medical history and honest with yourself about your lifestyle. Establish that your symptoms are really due to the menopause first. If you feel generally tense and tired and are under a lot of stress, try reducing the stress. If symptoms are interfering with your life and are definitely related to the menopause, such as hot flushes, and if you have tried unsuccessfully to alleviate the symptoms yourself and there are no medical reasons to prevent you taking HRT, then it might be worth trying for a short time. You can always stop if it does not help, or if you experience side-effects. Remember that deciding to use HRT to prevent osteoporosis requires persistence because longer-term treatment – at least five years – is usually recommended.

Paying attention to your diet and exercising are alternative and good preventative measures that you can take if you are premenopausal (see pages 104, 113).

WHERE CAN I GET HRT?

HRT is available on the NHS and can be prescribed by your family doctor or doctors at Well Woman or family planning clinics. There are also a few menopause clinics, funded by the NHS (see page 169 for addresses). If there are no such facilities near you and if you can afford it, private services are also available (see page 172).

First you need to find a doctor who is willing to explain the risks and benefits, and weigh them up with you. This could be your family doctor, a family planning doctor or a doctor at a Well Woman Clinic. It will also help to talk to friends and try to find someone who is sympathetic to your situation – avoid people with extreme views who dogmatically tell you what you must and must not do.

During, or soon after, the initial consultation, certain health checks should be carried out. Regular monitoring of your health is essential and follow-up appointments vary between every three months and once a year. It is vital that you report any irregular bleeding or symptoms, such as pains in your calves, chest or sudden shortness of breath, severe headaches or dizziness, jaundice or breast lumps. These could be signs of other illnesses and they should be investigated.

It is not advisable to start HRT when your periods are regular since your body is still producing adequate amounts of oestrogen, and too much oestrogen causes fluid retention, breast tenderness and irregular bleeding.

Doctors usually advise women to start HRT when their periods are already irregular.

HEALTH CHECKS YOU WILL NEED

Before starting HRT

- full medical history
- weight
- breast examination
- physical examination
- blood pressure
- internal vaginal examination
- cervical smear (every 3–5 years)★
- mammogram (every 2 years)★
- urine test for diabetes
- (sometimes) a blood test to determine your hormone levels

During HRT treatment

- blood pressure
- weight
- record any irregular bleeding
- breast examination
- internal examination

★ *If you are over 50 you should have these whether you are using HRT or not*

WHAT FORM OF HRT SHOULD I TAKE?

Again this is a personal decision, unless there are obvious medical advantages for you to use a particular method. Experts are currently advising against the use of synthetic hormones because of their side-effects. Natural oestrogens containing oestradiol are the safest forms of oestrogen, followed by conjugated oestrogens (containing oestradiol plus equine oestrogen). Women who are at risk of thrombosis or high blood pressure or who have liver problems should use patches or implants rather than pills. Because they bypass the liver these non-oral methods may well become the methods which are most popular in the future.

Progestogens should be taken for twelve to thirteen days each month to protect the lining of the womb. Some doctors recommend continued oestrogen throughout the month while others leave a five to seven-day gap of no treatment during the monthly bleed – it all depends on the product used. Ask your doctor to explain in detail about the type of oestrogen he or she recommends for you. Further information about the oestrogens available and the optimal doses can be found on page 161.

Some women do continue to use HRT for decades, however, most doctors recommend taking the smallest effective dose for the shortest possible time. For the treatment of hot flushes this would be for between six months and two years, and for the prevention of osteoporosis it is estimated that five years of treatment can be beneficial. Always remember that *the choice is yours*.

TYPES OF HRT

Pills

These contain oestrogen only (if you have had a hysterectomy) or combine oestrogen and progestogen (for the last 12–13 days) in calendar packs. Some doctors recommend stopping oestrogen for 5 days during the monthly bleeding.

Advantages:

Easy to take and dose can be quickly changed.

Disadvantages:

Some women get indigestion.

Creams

Usually recommended for vaginal dryness, they can be applied locally inside the vagina.

Advantages:

Small doses can be taken.

Disadvantages:

Not recommended for prevention of osteoporosis. They may not stop hot flushes because of the low dosage.

Patches

Small transparent plasters the size of a 10 pence piece are stuck on the lower half of the body, usually the hip or thigh. They contain oestrogen which is released into the blood stream.

Advantages:

Oestrogen does not pass through the liver, therefore the risks of side-effects are reduced. They provide a more constant level of oestrogen.

Disadvantages:

Patches need to be removed to a different spot at least twice a week (more often in hot weather) to avoid skin irritation. They can come off in the bath or when swimming. Progestogens still need to be taken by mouth for 12–13 days each month.

Implants

Tiny pellets containing oestrogen, which are the size of apple pips, are inserted under the skin of the buttock or groin. The effects last for up to 6 months.

Advantages:

You do not have to remember to take oestrogens and it does not pass through the liver.

Disadvantages:

The dose cannot be modified once the implant is inserted. They can be removed, but often with difficulty. Again a progestogen has to be taken by mouth for part of the month.

YOUR CHOICE

Ultimately any decision about whether to take HRT or not should depend mainly on whether you have severe hot flushes and night sweats or vaginal dryness, or a strong predisposition to develop osteoporosis in later life. Since many women are helped by alternative approaches, including relaxation, self-help groups and vitamins, which do not carry health risks, it surely makes sense to try these first. And since we know that preventative steps taken before the menopause can make a positive difference, you should make sure that you are well prepared too. This will remain sound advice for as long as there are possible health risks associated with HRT.

Weighing up these health risks also brings each of us face to face with fundamental questions. What is *normal* health? Should a section of the population be viewed as deficient and treated as such? Women have allowed the predominantly male medical world to provide the answers for too long – it is time for women to challenge some of the assumptions behind the treatments they are offered.

You must never forget that HRT is the product of a multi-billion dollar, multi-national pharmaceutical industry and that there are not such big profits to be made from self-help, relaxation or exercise. Obviously, from the perspective of the pharmaceutical industry, the more problems that HRT can be seen to solve the better.

Control over our bodies is often equated with freedom of choice but, paradoxically, for many women the development of reproductive technologies has increased the capacity of others to control our lives. Today it is even more important that women are informed enough to make their *own* choices about how they deal with the menopause.

You may believe that the menopause is a normal stage of a woman's life, and put your faith in natural methods of alleviating the worst symptoms. But if you do have a bad time and if, having considered the pros and cons, you decide that HRT is the answer for you, you should not feel guilty or think that you are a failure. Women face similar dilemmas when planning for childbirth and many, who keenly attend natural childbirth antenatal classes, decide that they do need to resort to epidurals, forceps or caesarean births for the sake of their child's and sometimes their own health. Similarly, in one menopause workshop I attended, a few women initially felt inadequate because they had found their menopause more difficult to deal with than others who had sailed through it. We need to accept our differences and respect each other's decisions about treatment, so long as these are made with a clear understanding of the issues involved and the available alternatives.

9

A Positive Future

With a third of their lives ahead of them, many women approaching the menopause can look forward to a future offering more time and more choices. Jokes abound about the so-called mid-life crisis, a stage that men seem to hit at around 40, but it does everyone good to take stock of past achievements and disappointments, while contemplating future desires and objectives.

You might want to question some of the assumptions that exist about how older women should behave and how they should occupy themselves. For example, shouldn't you complain when you are discriminated against, and should women necessarily become less active and more isolated with age?

As most women in their fifties and sixties do not generally regard themselves as old, it is difficult for them to identify with the negative stereotypes of older women. Winnie, 55, and Jean, 59, are looking forward to an early retirement:

I know that everyone says that your body ages around

you but inside you feel young at heart. Well it's certainly true for me.

In my opinion life gets better! I'm more confident, less troubled by silly anxieties, and I care less what people think. When I retire next year I'm planning to do all those things I haven't had time for so far.

Neither is this stage of life necessarily associated with ill-health – most women in their fifties and sixties are in reasonable health. And you can keep yourself fit and healthy by keeping active and eating well.

Women like Winnie and Jean represent an ever increasing proportion of the population. They are not 'old' in the traditional, negative sense – dependent, ill, inactive – and so they are difficult even for experts to define. Bernice Neugarten, a North American psychologist and an authority on ageing, describes this stage as 'young-old'; Dr Eric Midwinter, director of the Centre for Policy on Ageing in the UK, uses the term 'the Third Age' to describe the stage of active independence and retirement. Work and mainstream family life constitutes the Second Age; the First Age is childhood and education, while the Fourth Age refers to dependence and decline. He believes that:

The Third Age should be lengthy and socially profitable, a phase of happy self-redirection, and the Fourth Age should be postponed as long as possible and become a quiet brief spell of dependence.

What choices might you face? You might want to continue your career or change direction. Some people want to work less hard so that they have time to pursue more leisure activities. Phased retirement is becoming more popular so this could well be a possibility if you want to, and if you can afford it.

However, if you have felt unfulfilled during your working life or if you feel just ready for a change, the 1990s promise more opportunities for women. Because of the predicted skills shortage within Britain as the number of young people joining the workforce declines, leading employers, such as the high street banks, are encouraging older women to return to work. Three quarters of all new jobs created during the 1990s are expected to be filled by women. Many, of course, will be part-time and low-grade jobs but such a huge shift in the composition of the national labour force is bound to open doors previously closed to women. This could be the time to develop new skills or to demonstrate your existing abilities to the full.

Sheila, who is 42, has a high-powered job in advertising:

> Looking ahead I would like to do something different – I don't want to continue at this pace for ever. I'd really like to open a small restaurant with some friends. Now I think that people accept that they make chops and changes in their working lives.

Jo, 58, has always wanted to work with animals, but did not have the opportunity or the time to follow her interests. She spent nine years looking after her mother, who died last year, and took occasional part-time work purely for the money:

> I go to help out at the local animal refuge three days a week. I'm learning all the time about the practical

aspects of caring for the animals, as well as their different natures and instincts. Soon I'll be able to work as an assistant. It doesn't pay very well but my mother left me some money, and I love it.

For women who have spent many years looking after children, mid-life can represent a new-found freedom. Because families tend to be much smaller than they were in the past, parental obligation is often discharged more quickly. And so for many women the Third Age is the time when they discover the joy of leisure. This was the case for Mary, 67, who describes life after the menopause:

It's the first time since starting a family that you can be selfish without feeling guilty. I notice the freedom, for example, of only having yourself to dry after swimming! I can come and go as I please and have room in the house to leave *my own* hobbies lying around.

Katie, who lost her husband five years ago, has picked up the pieces and is now enjoying a new independence:

I have made a circle of friends who are roughly my age – it was my saviour. We go out together several times a week shopping, dancing or swimming. I have also started going abroad for my holidays – something I've never done before. But I do miss not having a car – I don't drive.

For Margaret, 58, grandparenthood brings particular pleasure:

What is good about this stage of life? Picking up the

wonderful relationship with my grandchildren that I had with my own grandparents.

The advantages of the postmenopausal years also include the opportunity to improve relationships. With fewer commitments in terms of work or childcare, many women with partners find that it becomes easier to have more equal roles. Men often want to spend more time being domestic, especially when they have retired. It is a time to reassess roles and make changes to suit your needs.

If you have resentments about the past, or unfulfilled wishes, try to channel them into something that you can achieve. Amy had for many years harboured resentment towards her husband because she felt that he avoided challenges and was unambitious:

> I realise now that it was his decision, and that I was probably wanting him to succeed for both of us. Now I've started an Open University degree and, although it's difficult at times, I feel good about myself and I have more respect for my husband.

Many women discover that their relationships with other women deepen and that lasting friendships develop. Whatever your circumstances, there are likely to be many other women in a similar situation. Several groups and organisations for older women are beginning to find a voice and are campaigning for better health and social services. For details of organisations and support groups see pages 165–7.

If you are one of the generation of women now looking ahead to the menopause and the years that follow, you are at an historic crossroads. You have fought for and witnessed many positive changes for women in the second half of the twentieth century. Now you can attempt to change attitudes and to prepare for the future – you can have an easier menopause and a more rewarding Third Age than previous generations.

The menopause is one of life's milestones – use it to plan for a positive future. Gwyn puts it in perspective:

Most of my friends look back on their menopause with a sense of affection and humour. All are pleased to have come through it and wouldn't go back to having periods. Women shouldn't dread the menopause – it's just a stage and life goes on.

Information and Resources

THE HUNTER MENOPAUSE PROJECT

To find out what ordinary women really experience during the menopause I approached over 1000 women who were voluntarily attending an ovarian screening facility at King's College Hospital, London. Eight hundred and fifty agreed to complete a 5 page questionnaire on women's health. The *Women's Health Questionnaire* was carefully designed to elicit an unbiased picture of the health and well-being of women aged between 45 and 65. It covered a range of areas including general health and mood, use of medical services, as well as attitudes to and experience of the menopause.

The women came mainly from South East England and their average age was 52 years (ranging from 45 to 65). The majority (81%) were married and two-thirds were working outside the home, either full-time or part-time. They were similar to the general population of women living in South East England in terms of social class, employment and marital status. None of the women contacted had ovarian cancer and they were not unusually health conscious.

Two-thirds had already had their menopause, while 23% were perimenopausal. A smaller proportion (16%) had not yet reached the menopause. Of all the women, 12% had had a hysterectomy and 8% were taking HRT at the time. Comparison of these groups of women provided full details about their health and the impact of the menopause.

But to get a clearer picture some of the women, who were premenopausal, were followed for 3 years until a proportion of them (36) became menopausal. With this additional information it was possible to clarify which changes are due to the menopause and which were associated with ageing, stress or other events. In addition it was possible to predict who might be more likely to have particular problems during this life stage.

The research was carried out on a part-time basis between 1983 and 1988, while I was employed as a clinical psychologist by the Camberwell Health Authority.

HRT PREPARATIONS
Pills

Trade Name	Type of Oestrogen	Daily Dose
Hormonin	Natural – oestradiol + ostrone + oestriol	
Progynova	Natural – oestradiol valerate	1–3mgs of
Questrin	Natural – oestriol	oestradiol
Premarin	Conjugated – equilin + dihyrdroequilin + ostrone	0.625 mgs or 1.25 mgs
Dienoestrol	Synthetic – dienoestrol	
Ethinyloestradiol	Synthetic – ethinyloestradiol	15 mcgs

Plus progestogen for 12 – 13 days each month orally

Progestogens

Noriday	Synthetic – Norethisterone	1–3 mgs
Provera	Synthetic – Medroxyprogesterone	
Duphaston	Synthetic – Dydrogesterone	
Neogest	Synthetic – Norgestrel	0.15–0.5 mgs

Combined oestrogen and progestogen packs

Menophase	Synthetic – Mestranol + Norethisterone (continuous oestrogen, 13 days progestogen)
Prempak	Conjugated – Premarin (as above) + Norgestrel (21 days oestrogen + progestogen, 7 days no treatment)
Prempak C	Conjugated as above (continuous oestrogen, 12 days low dose progestogen)
Cycloprogynova	Natural – oestradiol valerate (21 days oestrogen, 10 days progestogen, 7 days no treatment)

Vaginal creams

Ovestin	Natural – oestriol	1–3 mgs
Premarin	Conjugated – as above	

Implants

Oestradiol	Natural – oestradiol	25, 50 or 100 mgs every 6 months

Patches

Estraderm	Natural – oestradiol

SELF HELP GROUPS AND ORGANISATIONS

MENOPAUSE GROUPS (UK)

For information about menopause self help groups in your area, the following organisations should be able to help:
Women's Health Information Centre
52, Featherstone Street, London EC1 (01 251 6580)

Women's Health Concern,
17, Earl's Terrace, London W8 6LP

Your Community Health Council
(see telephone directory or 01 272 5459)

Your Health Education Unit
(see telephone directory or 01 637 1881)

Your local Health Centre, Well Woman Clinic or Family Planning Clinic
(see telephone directory)

WIRES (for local women's groups)
P.O. Box 20, Oxford. (0865 240991)

Mid-Life Centre, Birmingham Settlement

318, Summer Lane, Birmingham B19 3RL (021 359 3562 Tuesday and Thursday)

Although there is not yet a national network of menopause support groups, several groups and workshops do exist. The following are examples of established menopause or midlife support groups set up for women locally. They are happy to be contacted:

Women's Midlife Group
Victoria Health Centre, Glasshouse Street, Nottingham (0602 480500)

Well Woman Centre
Trinity Community Centre, Middle Street, Lancaster (0524 63760)

Well Woman Centre
Iris Adair, 3, Botanic Avenue, Belfast, Northern Ireland (0232 324914)

Hampstead Community Health Council
10, New End, Hampstead, London NW3 (01 794 9953)

Well Women Project
Shoreditch Health Centre, 210 Kingsland Road, London E2

The Amarant Trust (80, Lambeth Road, London SE1 7PW; 01 928 5633) is in the process of establishing a national network of Amarant support groups. Their aim is to provide information about HRT, increase access to it by encouraging GPs to prescribe HRT and to raise funds for research into HRT and for more menopause clinics so that HRT will be more widely available. The groups also aim to offer advice and support on midlife issues. Several such groups have begun. For example:

Amarant Support Group
Berwick on Tweed (0289 306008)

Amarant Trust Support Group for Menopausal Problems
9, Christopher Close, Yeovil, Somerset

WOMEN'S HEALTH AND SUPPORT GROUPS (UK)

Women's Health Information Centre
52, Featherstone Street, London EC1 (01 251 6580)

National Osteoporosis Society
PO Box 10, Barton Meade House, Radstock, Bath BA3 3YB

Hysterectomy Support Groups
c/o Ann Webb, 11 Henryson Road, London SE4 1HL
Judy Vaughn, Riverdell, Warren Way, Lower Heswall, Wirral, L10 9HV (051 345 3162)

Endometriosis Society
c/o Alisa Irvine, 65 Holmdene Avenue, Herne Hill, London SE24 9LD

Women's National Cancer Control Campaign
1 South Audley Street, London W1Y 5DQ (01 499 7532)

Drugs, Alcoholism, Women Nationally (DAWN)
146 Victoria Street, London EC4

Alcohol Concern
305 Grays Inn Road, London WC1X 8QF (01 833 3471)

Release
169 Commercial Street, London EC1 6BW (01 377 5905)
(For self-help network for tranquilliser withdrawal.)

Women's Sexuality Groups
Redwood Women's Training Association, 83 Fordwych Road, London NW2 (01 452 9261)

National Association for the Childless
318 Summer Lane, Birmingham B19 3RL (021 359 4887)

Older Feminists Network
c/o A Woman's Place, Hungerford House, Victoria Embankment, London WC2 (01 836 6081)

COUNSELLING AND THERAPY (UK)

Albany Women's Advice and Counselling Service
The Albany, Deptford, London SE8 (01 692 6268)

Bereavement Counselling
Contact local Community Health Council or Social Services
Department or Clinical Psychology Department, or your local
MIND group (see below), or if you live in London contact:
The London Bereavement Projects Coordinating Group
c/o 68 Chalton Street, London NW1 (01 388 0241)

Birmingham Women's Counselling and Therapy Centre
43 Ladywood Middleway, Birmingham B16 8HA (021 455
8677)

British Association of Counselling
37A, Sheep Street, Rugby CV21 3BX (0788 78328)

CRUSE
Cruse House, 126 Sheen Road, Richmond, Surrey (01 940 4818)
(Provides advice and support for women whose partners have
died.)

MIND (National Association for Mental Health)
22, Harley Street, London W1N 2ED (01 637 0741)

Rape Crisis Centre
PO Box 69, London WC1 9NJ (01 837 1600 or 021 233 3122:
call to find out about your nearest centre)

Relate (formerly Marriage Guidance Council)
Head Office, Little Church Street, Rugby CV21 3AP (0788
73241)

Relaxation for Living
Dunesk, 29 Burwood Park Road, Walton-on-Thames, Surrey
KT12 5LH
(Produces leaflets and a correspondence course on relaxation.)

Samaritans
(See telephone directory, or telephone 01 283 8581)

Southampton Women's Counselling and Therapy Service
15, Harold Road, Shirley, Southampton

The Carer's National Association
29, Chilworth Mews, London W2 (01 724 7776)
(Provides information and support for those caring for an ill or
disabled relative.)

The National Association for Widows
54–57 Allison Street, Birmingham B5 5TH (021 643 8348)

Women's Therapy Centre
6 Manor Gardens, London N7 (01 263 6200)
(For individual therapy and groups dealing with eating
problems.)

Eating Disorders Association
Sackville Place, 44 Magdalen Street, Norwich, Norfolk (0603
621414)

ALTERNATIVE THERAPIES (UK)

Women's Natural Health Centre
c/o Kentish Town Women's Workshop, 169 Malden Road,
Kentish Town, London NW5 (01 267 5301)

Institute of Complementary Medicine
21 Portland Place, London W1N 3AF (01 636 9543)

British Homoeopathic Association
27a Devonshire Street, London W1N 1RJ

Society of Homoeopaths
47 Canada Grove, Bognor Regis, West Sussex PO21 1DW

The British Naturopathic and Osteopathic Association
Frazer House, 6 Netherhall Gardens, London NW3 5RR

National Institute of Medical Herbalists
41 Hatherley Road, Winchester, Hampshire SO22 6RR (0962 68776)

The British Acupuncture Association and Register
34 Alderney Street, London SW1V 4EU

SELF HELP GROUPS IN NEW ZEALAND

Women's Health Collective
63 Ponsonby Road, Auckland (764 506)

West Auckland Women's Centre
111 McLeod Road, Auckland (836 6381)

The Health Alternative for Women
PO Box 884, Christchurch (796 970)

Women's Health Collective
PO Box 9172, Wellington

Collective for Women
PO Box 8044, Dunedin (771 229)

SELF HELP GROUPS IN AUSTRALIA

For information about facilities in different states contact the Family Planning Association, or the department dealing with women's health in your state.

SELF HELP GROUPS IN THE USA

National Action Forum for Midlife and Older Women Inc,
Social and Behavioural Studies
N239, State University of New York, Stony Brook, New York
11794–4310

Climacteric Outreach
Centre for Climacteric Studies, University of Florida, 901 NW
8th Avenue, Suite 5b, Gainsville, Florida 32601

SELF HELP GROUPS IN CANADA

A Friend Indeed (for women in the prime of their life)
4180 Wibon Avenue, Montreal, Quebec H4A 2TG
(provides a regular newsletter and contacts on all aspects of the
menopause and midlife)

Women's Health Education Network
PO Box 1276, Truro, Nova Scotia, B2N 5N2

MENOPAUSE CLINICS IN THE UK (NHS)

This list is not exclusive. You could also ask at your local
Well Woman Clinic, Family Planning Clinic or gynaecology
department of your local hospital.

Beckenham Hospital
379, Croydon Road, Beckenham, Kent (01 650 0125)

Women's Hospital
5, York Road, Birmingham (021 472 1377)

Birmingham and Midland Hospital for Women
Showall Green Lane, Sparkhill, Birmingham (021 772 1101)

Family Planning Clinic
Morley Street, Brighton, Sussex (0273 693600)

Dryburn Hospital
North Road, Durham (091 386 4911)

Royal Infirmary
Lauriston Place, Edinburgh (031 229 2477)

Queen Elizabeth Hospital
Gateshead, Tyne and Wear (091 487 8989)

Glasgow Royal Infirmary
Castle Street, Glasgow (041 552 3535)

Bone Metabolism Research Unit
Western Infirmary, Glasgow (041 339 8822)

Stobhill Hospital
Balornock Road, Glasgow (041 558 0111)

Family Planning Clinic
Hillingdon Hospital, Field Heath Road, Hillingdon, Middlesex
(0895 58191)

Airedale General Hospital
Steeton, Keighley, West Yorkshire (0535 52511 x 442)

Clarendon Wing, Leeds General Infirmary
Belmont Grove, Leeds (0532 432799 x 3886)

Royal Liverpool Hospital
Prescott Street, Liverpool (051 709 0141)

The London Hospital
Whitechapel, London E1 (01 377 7000 x 2030)

St. George's Medical School and Hospital
Blackshaw Road, London SW17 (01 672 1255 x 55960/1)

Dulwich Hospital
East Dulwich Grove, London SE5 (01 693 9236/3377)

Dept. of Obstetrics and Gynaecology, Guy's Hospital
London SE1 (01 955 5000)

Royal Free Hospital
Pond Street, London NW3 (01 794 0500 x 3868)

Menopause Clinic, King's College Hospital
Denmark Hill, London SE5 (01 733 0224)

Menopause Clinic, Queen Charlotte's Hospital
Goldhawk Road, London W6 (01 748 4666)

Samaritan Hospital for Women
Marylebone Road, London W1 (01 402 4211)

Queen Mary's Hospital
Roehampton, London SW15 (01 789 6611)

Gynaecology Outpatients Dept.,
North Manchester General Hospital
Crumpstall, Manchester (061 795 4567)

Montagu Hospital (Outpatients)
Adwick Road, Mexborough, South Yorkshire (0709 585171
x 219)

Dept. of Medicine, Newcastle General Hospital
Westgate Road, Newcastle upon Tyne (091 273 8811 x 22675)

Gynaecology Outpatient Dept., George Elliot Hospital
College Street, Nuneaton, Warwickshire (0203 384201)

Oldham and District General Hospital
Rochdale Road, Oldham, Lancashire (061 624 0420)

John Radcliffe Hospital, The Anderson Clinic, Headington,
Oxford (0865 64711 x 7795)

The Ella Gordon Centre, St. Mary's Hospital
Portsmouth, Hampshire (0705 866301)

Northern General Hospital
Gynaecology Dept., Herries Road, Sheffield (0742 232323)

Stafford District General Hospital
Weston Road, Stafford (0785 57731)

Woodhouse Park Clinic
Simonsway, Woodhouse Park, Wythenshaw, Manchester (061 437 4625)

If there is not a clinic in your area or if you wish to have private treatment the best way to find out about local facilities is to contact: The Amarant Trust, 80, Lambeth Road, London SE1. 01 928 5633.

MENOPAUSE CLINICS IN AUSTRALIA

University of Melbourne
Dept of Psychiatry, Clinical Sciences Block, c/o PO Royal Melbourne Hospital, Victoria 3050

The Royal Hospital for Women
Paddington, NSW.

Menopause Clinic
University of New South Wales, 4, Thorn Street, Edge Cliff, NSW 2027
For clinics in most states contact your Family Planning Association, details from: Australian Federation of Family Planning Associations, 70, George Street, Sydney, NSW 2000.

MENOPAUSE CLINICS IN NEW ZEALAND

Family Planning Clinics offer counselling and advice and will be able to recommend a gynaecologist specialising in the menopause if you need to see one. Educational courses are also organised by the Family Planning Association. To find out more contact: Auckland 796 182, Christchurch 790 514 or Wellington 849 744.

MENOPAUSE CLINICS IN THE USA

Most gynaecologists provide health care and treatment for menopausal problems and some states have centres specialising in menopause and midlife.

Midlife Challenge
Marsha Flint, Dept. of Anthropology, Montclair State College, Upper Montclair, New Jersey 07043

Centre for Climacteric Studies
University of Florida, 901 NW 8th Avenue, Suite 5b, Gainsville, Florida 32601

Yale University Health Services
Division of Mental Hygiene, 17 Hillhouse Avenue, New Haven, Connecticut 06510

School of Medicine
Department of Obstetrics and Gynaecology, Center for Health Sciences, Los Angeles, California 90024

The Michigan Center for Diagnosis and Treatment of Osteoporosis
35000 Schoolcraft Road, Livonia, Michigan 48150

MENOPAUSE CLINICS IN CANADA

Department of Obstetrics and Gynaecology,
University of Saskatchewan, Sas S7N 9X0

Department of Obstetrics, Gynaecology and Medicine
339, Windermere Road, London, Ontario N6A 5A5

Mature Woman Clinic
Toronto General Hospital, Toronto, Ontario

FURTHER READING

Chapter 1

Our Bodies Ourselves, Ed. Angela Phillips and Jill Rakusen (Penguin 1978).

The Menopause, Jill Rakusen (Health Education Authority 1989).

Why Suffer? Periods and their Problems, Lynda Birke and Katy Gardner (Virago 1979).

Hysterectomy, Lorraine Dennerstein, Carl Wood and Graham Burrows (Oxford University Press 1982).

Women on Hysterectomy, Nicki Henriques and Ann Dickson (Thorsons 1986).

Chapter 2

Female Cycles, Paula Weideger (The Women's Press 1978).

Look Me in the Eye: Older Women Ageing and Ageism, Barbara MacDonald and Cynthia Rich (Spinsters Ink, San Francisco 1984).

Ageing for Beginners, Mary Stott (Basil Blackwell 1981).

Chapter 3

Prime Time, Helen Franks (Pan 1981).

The Menopause Leaflet, from Women's Health and Reproductive Rights Information Centre (54–56 Featherstone Street, London EC1Y 8RT).

Women's Experience of Sex, Sheila Kitzinger (Penguin 1985).

The Mirror Within, Ann Dickson (Quartet 1982).

Get a Better Nights Sleep, Ian Oswald and Kirstine Adam (Positive Health Guide, MacDonald Optima 1983).

Brittle Bones and the Calcium Crisis, Kathleen Mayes (Grapevine 1987).

Chapter 4

Dealing with Depression, Kathy Nairne and Gerrilyn Smith (Women's Press 1984).

Depression: The Way Out of Your Prison, Dorothy Rowe (Routledge 1983).

In Our Own Hands. A Book of Self Help Therapy, Sheila Ernst and Lucy Goodison (Women's Press 1981).

A Woman in Your Own Right, Ann Dickson (Quartet Books 1982).

The Courage to Grieve, Judy Tatelbaum (Heinemann 1981).

The Experience of Infertility, Naomi Pfeffer and Anne Woollett (Virago 1983).

Chapter 5

The Female Malady, Elaine Showalter (Virago 1987).

For Her Own Good: 150 years of the experts' advice to women, Barbara Ehrenreich and Deirdre English (Pluto Press 1979).

The Women's History of the World, Rosalind Miles (1988).

Chapter 6

Overcoming the Menopause Naturally, Caroline Shreeve (Arrow 1986).

The Right Way to Eat to Feel Good or Even Better, Miriam Polunin (Dent 1984).

Fat is a Feminist Issue, Susie Orbach (Arrow 1984).

Stand Tall! The informed woman's guide to preventing osteoporosis, Morris Notelovitz and Marsha Ware (Triad, Florida 1982).

Chapter 7

Stress and Relaxation, Jane Madders (Positive Health Guide, Dunitz 1979).

The Menopause: A Woman's View, Ann Dickson and Nicki Henriques (Thorsons 1987).

Menopause, A Time for Positive Change, Judi Fairlie, Jayne Nelson and Ruth Popplestone (Blandford Press 1987).

Natural Healing in Gynecology, Rina Nissim (Pandora 1986).

The Alternative Health Guide, Brian Inglis and Ruth West (Michael Joseph 1983).

Chapter 8

The Menopause, John Studd and Margaret Thom (Hamlyn 1981).

Life Change, Barbara Evans (Pan Books 1979).

No Change, Wendy Cooper (Arrow 1983).

Menopause: A Positive Approach, Rosetta Reitz (Unwin Hyman 1985).

HRT and You, Kate de Selincourt (Booklet published by the Independent newspaper 1989).

These books cover a range of views about HRT.

Breast Cancer: A Guide to its Detection and Treatment, Carolyn Faulder (Virago 1982).

Chapter 9

Returning to Work: Education and Training for Women, Women Returning to Work Network (Longmans).

It's Never Too Late: A Practical Guide to Continuing Education for Women of all Ages, Joan Perkin (Impact Books 1984).

The Time of Your Life: A Handbook for Retirement, Aleda Erskine (Health Education Council 1981).

REFERENCES

Introduction

1. Kaufert PA (1984) Women and their health in the middle years, *Social Science and Medicine* 18, 3, 279–281.
2. Mckinlay SM and Mckinlay JB (1986) Health status and health care utilization by menopausal women. In Notelovitz M and Van Keep P (Eds) *The Climacteric in Perspective*, MTP Press Ltd., Lancaster.
3. Holte A and Mikkelsen A (1982) Menstrual coping style, social background and climacteric symptoms, *Psychiatry and Social Science*, 2, 41–45.
4. Hunter MS (1988) Psychological and somatic experience of the climacteric and postmenopause: predicting individual differences and helpseeking behaviour, Phd Thesis, university of London.

Chapter 1

1. Van Keep PA et al (1983) Hysterectomy in European countries, *Maturitas*, 5, 2, 69–77.
2. Parlee MB (1978) Psychological aspects of the climacteric in women, *Psychiatric Opinion*, 15, 9, 36–40.
3. Dennerstein L and Ryan M (1982) Psychosocial and emotional sequelae of hysterectomy, *Journal of Psychosomatic Obstetrics and Gynaecology*, 1–2, 81–86.
4. Wallace L (1984) Psychological preparation for gynaecological surgery. In Broome A and Wallace L (Eds) *Psychology and Gynaecological Problems*, Tavistock, London.
5. Kaufert PA et al (1987) Defining the menopause: the impact of longitudinal data, *Maturitas*, 9, 217–226.
6. Voda AM (1981) The climacteric hot flush, *Maturitas*, 3, 73–90.

Chapter 2

1. Lock M (1986) Ambiguities of ageing: Japanese experience and perceptions of the menopause, *Culture, Medicine and Psychiatry*, 10, 23–46. Cites Kaufert's data.

2. Van Keep PA (1970) *The menopause; a study of attitudes of women in six European countries*. International Health Foundation, Geneva.

3. Neugarten BL et al (1963) Women's attitudes to the menopause, *Vita Humana*, 6, 140–151.

4. Cowan G et al (1985) Medical perceptions of menopausal symptoms, *Psychology of Women Quarterly*, 9(1), 3–14.

5. Leiblum SR and Swartzman LS (1986) Women's attitudes to the menopause; an update, *Maturitas*, 8, 47–56.

6. Mitchell J (1974) *Psychoanalysis and Feminism*, Penguin, London.

7. Chasseguet-Smirgel J (1970) *Female Sexuality, New Psychoanalytic Views*, Maresfield Library, London.

8. Smith J (1989) *The Genesis of Misogynies*, Faber, London.

9. Morgan F (1989) *A Misogynist's Source Book*, Jonathan Cape, London.

Chapter 3

1. Kaufert PA (1984) Women and their health in the middle years, *Social Science and Medicine* 18, 3, 279–281.

2. Mckinlay SM and Mckinlay JB (1986) Health status and health care utilization by menopausal women. In Notelovitz M and Van Keep P (Eds) *The Climacteric in Perspective*, MTP Press Ltd., Lancaster.

3. Holte A (1987) The Norweigan Menopausal Project, paper presented at 5th International Menopause Congress, Sorrento, Italy.

4. Hunter MS et al (1986) Relationships between psychological symptoms, somatic complaints and menopausal status, *Maturitas*, 8, 217–28.

5. Ballinger S et al (1979) Life stresses and depression in the menopause, *Maturitas*, 1, 191–199.

6. Kinsey AC et al (1963) *Sexual Behaviour in the Human Female*, Pocket Books, New York.

7. Bungay GT et al (1980) Study of symptoms in middle life with special reference to the menopause, *British Medical Journal*, ii, 181–183.

8. Hite S (1988) *The Hite Report*, Pandora Press.

9. Bancroft J (1983) *Human Sexuality and its Problems*, Churchill Livingstone, Edinburgh.

10. Bachmann GA et al (1984) Sexual expression and its determinants in postmenopausal women, *Maturitas*, 6, 19–29.

11. Ballinger CB et al (1987) Hormone profiles and psychological symptoms in perimenopausal women, *Maturitas*, 9, 235–251.

12. Dow MGT and Gallagher J (1989) A controlled study of combined hormonal and psychological treatment for sexual unresponsiveness in women, *British Journal of Clinical Psychology*, 28, 201–212.

13. Vessey M and Hunt K (1988) The menopause, hormone replacement therapy and cardiovascular disease. In Studd JJ and Whitehead MI, *The Menopause*, Blackwell Sci. Publ. London (p. 190).

14. Hunt K et al (1987) Long-term surveillance of mortality and cancer incidence in women receiving hormone replacement therapy, *British Journal of Obstetrics and Gynaecology*, 94, 620–635.

15. Wilson PWF et al (1985) Postmenopausal oestrogen use, cigarette smoking and cardiovascular morbidity in women over 50. The Framingham Study, *New England Journal of Medicine*, 313, 1038–43.

Chapter 4

1. Ballinger CB et al (1987) Hormone profiles and psychological symptoms in perimenopausal women, *Maturitas*, 9, 235–251.

2. Coope J (1981) Is oestrogen therapy effective in the treatment of menopausal depression? *Journal of the Royal College of General Practitioners*, 31, 134–140.

3. Utian WH (1972) The mental tonic effect of oestrogens administered to oophorectomized females, *South African Medical Journal*, 46, 1079–82.

Chapter 5

1. Flint M (1975) The menopause: reward or punishment? *Psychosomatics*, 16, 161–163.

2. Lock M (1986) Ambiguities of ageing: Japanese experience and perceptions of the menopause, *Culture, Medicine and Psychiatry*, 10, 23–46.

3. Beyenne YC (1986) Cultural significance and physiological manifestations of the menopause, a biocultural analysis, *Culture, Medicine and Psychiatry*, 10, 47–71.

4. Wilbush J (1979) La menespausie – the birth of a syndrome, *Maturitas*, 1, 145–151.

5. Showalter E (1985) *The Female Malady*, Virago, London.

6. Deutsch H (1945) *The Psychology of Women*, Vol. 2. Grune and Stratton, New York.

7. McCrea FB (1983) The politics of the menopause: the 'discovery' of a deficiency disease. *Social Problems*, 31, 1, 110–122.

8. Phillips A and Rakusen J (Eds) (1978) *Our Bodies Ourselves – a health book for and by women*, Penguin, England.

9. Reitz R (1981) *Menopause – a positive approach*, Unwin Paperbacks.

Chapter 6

1. Notelovitz M (1988) Non-hormonal management of the menopause. In Studd JJ and Whitehead MI, *The Menopause*, Blackwell, London (p. 107).

2. Beverly MC et al (1989) Local bone mineral response to brief exercise that stresses the skeleton, *British Medical Journal*, Vol 299 22 July 233–235.

3. Smith EL et al (1981) Physical activity and calcium modalities for bone mineral increase in aged women, *Medicine and Science in Sports and Exercise*, 13, 60–64.

4. Stewart M and Stewart A (1987) *Beat PMT Through Diet*, Ebury Press.

5. Notelovitz M (1988) Non-hormonal management of the menopause. In Studd JJ and Whitehead MI, *The Menopause*, Blackwell, London (p. 107).

6. *New Health*, Nov. 1983 p. 104.

7. Notelovitz M (1988) Non-hormonal management of the menopause. In Studd JJ and Whitehead MI, *The Menopause*, Blackwell, London (p. 113).

Chapter 8

1. Whitehead MI and Studd JJ (1988) Selection of patients for treatment: which therapy and for how long? In Studd JJ and Whitehead MI, *The menopause*, Blackwell, London (p. 126).

2. Brinton LA et al (1986) Menopausal oestrogens and breast cancer risk; an expanded case–control study, *British Journal of Cancer*, 54, 825–832.

Index

Also Available from Pandora Press

The Hite Report *Shere Hite*	£5.99☐
The Midwife Challenge *Sheila Kitzinger* (ed)	£6.95☐
Drugs in Pregnancy and Childbirth *Judy Priest*	£5.99☐
Miscarriage *Christine Moulder*	£5.99☐
Being Fat is Not a Sin *Shelley Bovey*	£4.99☐
Living with a Drinker *Mary Wilson*	£4.99☐
Infertility *Renate D Klein* (ed)	£4.95☐
Natural Healing in Gynaecology *Rina Nissim*	£4.95☐
Birth and Our Bodies *Paddy O'Brien*	£4.50☐
Your Life After Birth *Paddy O'Brien*	£4.95☐
Women's Health: A *Spare Rib* Reader *Sue O'Sullivan* (ed)	£5.95☐
The Politics of Breastfeeding *Gabrielle Palmer*	£6.95☐
Motherhood; What It Does To Your Mind *Jane Price*	£4.95☐
Until They Are Five *Angela Phillips*	£4.99☐
Women and the AIDS Crisis *Diane Richardson*	£3.95☐
On Your Own: A Guide to Independent Living *Jean Shapiro*	£6.95☐
The Heroin Users *Tom Stewart*	£5.95☐

All these books are available at your local bookshop or newsagent or can be ordered direct by post. Just tick the titles you want and fill in the form below.

Name_____

Address_____

_____

_____

Write to Unwin Hyman Cash Sales, PO Box 11, Falmouth Cornwall TR10 9ED.

Please enclose remittance to the value of the cover price plus: U.K. 80p for the first book plus 20p for each additional book ordered to a maximum charge of £2.00.

BFPO: 80p for the first book plus 20p for each additional book.

OVERSEAS INCLUDING EIRE: £1.50 for the first book plus £1.00 for the second book and 30p for each additional book.

Pandora Press reserve the right to show new retail prices on covers, which may differ from those previously advertised in the text and elsewhere. Postage rates are also subject to revision.